T0260124

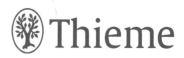

Handbook of Pediatric Orthopaedics

Third Edition

Paul D. Sponseller, MD, MBA
Sponseller Professor and Head,
Division of Pediatric Orthopaedics
Johns Hopkins Medical Institutions
Baltimore, Maryland

Thieme
New York • Stuttgart • Delhi • Rio de Janeiro

Thieme Medical Publishers, Inc.
333 Seventh Avenue
New York, New York 10001

Executive Editor: William Lamsback
Managing Editor: J. Owen Zurhellen
Director, Editorial Services: Mary Jo Casey
Production Editor: Sean Woznicki
International Production Director: Andreas Schabert
Editorial Director: Sue Hodgson
International Marketing Director: Fiona Henderson
International Sales Director: Louisa Turrell
Director of Institutional Sales: Adam Bernacki
Senior Vice President and Chief Operating Officer:
    Sarah Vanderbilt
President: Brian D. Scanlan
Front Cover Illustration: Purva Chimurkar

Library of Congress Cataloging-in-Publication Data

Names: Sponseller, Paul D., author.
Title: Handbook of pediatric orthopaedics / Paul D.
Sponseller.
Other titles: Handbook of pediatric orthopedics
Description: Third edition. | New York : Thieme,
[2019] | Preceded by Handbook of pediatric
orthopedics / Paul D. Sponseller. 2nd ed. c2011.
| Includes bibliographical references and index.
Identifiers: LCCN 2018051040| ISBN 9781626234314
(pbk. : alk. paper) | ISBN 9781626234321 (e-book)
Subjects: | MESH: Orthopedics | Child | Infant |
Handbooks
Classification: LCC RD732.3.C48 | NLM WS 39 |
DDC 618.92/7–dc23 LC record available at
https://lccn.loc.gov/2018051040

Copyright © 2020 by Thieme Medical Publishers, Inc.

Thieme Publishers New York
333 Seventh Avenue, New York, NY 10001 USA
+1 800 782 3488, customerservice@thieme.com

Thieme Publishers Stuttgart
Rüdigerstrasse 14, 70469 Stuttgart, Germany
+49 [0]711 8931 421, customerservice@thieme.de

Thieme Publishers Delhi
A-12, Second Floor, Sector-2, Noida-201301
Uttar Pradesh, India
+91 120 45 566 00, customerservice@thieme.in

Thieme Publishers Rio de Janeiro, Thieme Publicações
Ltda.
Edifício Rodolpho de Paoli, 25º andar
Av. Nilo Peçanha, 50 – Sala 2508,
Rio de Janeiro 20020-906 Brasil
+55 21 3172-2297 / +55 21 3172-1896
www.thiemerevinter.com.br

Cover design: Thieme Publishing Group
Typesetting by Thomson Digital, India

Printed in Germany by CPI books, Leck

5 4 3 2 1

ISBN 978-1-62623-431-4

Also available as an e-book:
eISBN 978-1-62623-432-1

Important note: Medicine is an ever-changing science undergoing continual development. Research and clinical experience are continually expanding our knowledge, in particular our knowledge of proper treatment and drug therapy. Insofar as this book mentions any dosage or application, readers may rest assured that the authors, editors, and publishers have made every effort to ensure that such references are in accordance with **the state of knowledge at the time of production of the book.**

Nevertheless, this does not involve, imply, or express any guarantee or responsibility on the part of the publishers in respect to any dosage instructions and forms of applications stated in the book. **Every user is requested to examine carefully** the manufacturers' leaflets accompanying each drug and to check, if necessary in consultation with a physician or specialist, whether the dosage schedules mentioned therein or the contraindications stated by the manufacturers differ from the statements made in the present book. Such examination is particularly important with drugs that are either rarely used or have been newly released on the market. Every dosage schedule or every form of application used is entirely at the user's own risk and responsibility. The authors and publishers request every user to report to the publishers any discrepancies or inaccuracies noticed. If errors in this work are found after publication, errata will be posted at www.thieme.com on the product description page.

Some of the product names, patents, and registered designs referred to in this book are in fact registered trademarks or proprietary names even though specific reference to this fact is not always made in the text. Therefore, the appearance of a name without designation as proprietary is not to be construed as a representation by the publisher that it is in the public domain.

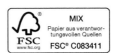

I dedicate this third edition to the students, residents, and fellows who have continuously inspired me and who enabled me to look at problems in new ways.

Contents

Foreword

Dear Readers:

It is always a pleasure to share a good book. "Check this great section," or "I especially found that illustration useful," or "Helpful summary on page X" are great phrases to say when sharing a reference. I used those phrases in abundance while reading this book, and I am especially pleased to recommend the third edition of the *Handbook of Pediatric Orthopaedics* by Paul D. Sponseller. As with previous editions, this third edition is a fantastic resource for orthopaedists, orthopaedic trainees, medical students, nurses, and advanced practitioners who care for pediatric orthopaedic patients. It compiles volumes of knowledge and important pediatric orthopaedic data and boils them down to the important points in an easy-to-read and easy-to-reference handbook. This edition is arranged in a chapter format similar to that of the previous editions and has updated content. Importantly, the book allows quick reference in the clinic setting, on rounds, and for case learning and planning and remains a great resource.

"Check this great section": Normal growth and development are very well described and provide a strong base for learning in the sections that follow. This section is full of useful tables and references. Quickly answer the often-asked clinic question "How tall will my child be?" and share rotation data for the lower extremity with families. New in this edition, check the enhanced section on gait analysis.

"I especially found this figure useful": Simple illustrative figures include the common sites and types of bone lesions, the Lenke classification of idiopathic scoliosis curves, and types and associations of tibial bowing. This third edition contains new, useful figures, such as additional Legg–Calvé–Perthes disease illustrations and a great fracture line map of triplane ankle fractures.

"Helpful summary on": There are great summaries on topics such as the management of hip dysplasia, the types of muscular disorders in pediatric orthopaedics, the gross motor functional classification system in cerebral palsy, and skeletal dysplasia and syndromes. New helpful summaries in this third edition include an expanded discussion of femur fractures and updated imaging parameters for many common pediatric orthopaedic conditions.

I find this handbook full of practical information for pediatric orthopaedics and look forward to referring to it with my residents and fellows. Congratulations and thank you once again to Dr. Sponseller: our trainees, practitioners, and our patients will benefit from your book. Again, readers, I am certain you will find the great sections, the especially useful illustrations, and the helpful summaries. I am very pleased to share this good book with you.

Michelle S. Caird, MD
Larry S. Matthews Collegiate Professor of Orthopaedic Surgery
Chief of Pediatric Orthopaedic Surgery
University of Michigan
Ann Arbor, Michigan

Preface

Effective care in pediatric orthopaedics builds on principles and on technical skills. Often we also need to refer to data and standards. In the process of teaching children's orthopaedics, I have tried to refine and condense information that is essential for the practice of our specialty. I gathered these "pearls" into a practical handbook that is complete yet concise, and the first and second editions were well received. Hence this fully revised and updated third edition. This handbook is not meant to provide definitive coverage of individual problems or theoretical principles. Rather, its purpose is to provide factual information for quick reference.

The first chapter, Anatomy and Normal Development in Children, gives norms for osseous development, motor development, innervation, and growth patterns and predictions. There are many exciting new guidelines for assessing growth at the pelvis, foot, and hand, which are described here. Much information on gait and its analysis is also new. Chapters 2, 3, and 4 about disorders of skeletal growth and development have been expanded and provide concise, practical information on even more of the common conditions we treat. This includes imaging parameters and clinical standards for treatment. Chapter 5, Skeletal Syndromes and Systemic Disorders in Pediatric Orthopaedics, has been improved with the newest knowledge in this fast-changing field. Chapter 6, Neuromuscular Disorders in Pediatric Orthopaedics, covers cerebral palsy, myelodsplasia, spinal muscular atrophy, and recent advances in their treatment. Next is an important chapter on pediatric trauma, with updates on forearm and femur fractures (Chapter 7), followed by Chapter 8, Normal Values and Medications, which provides a useful reference on the most common lab values (with age-related changes) and drugs. The last chapter, on common procedures, provides a how-to in bulleted form to walk the reader through blocks, traction, special casts, aspiration, and arthrograms.

I have filled this handbook with information that I use in the daily practice of pediatric orthopaedics. There is something in it for those at all levels. I trust you will find it rewarding.

Paul D. Sponseller, MD, MBA
Baltimore, Maryland

Acknowledgments

I thank those students, residents, and fellows whom I have been privileged to help train: their insights stimulate me to continuously question what might otherwise be taken for granted. I thank my family—Amy, Ruth, Matt, and Nina—for their inspiration. The careful editing of J. Owen Zurhellen IV, and the clear, concise line drawings by Hong Cui, MD, have made this book possible. Finally, the innovative front cover art by Purva Chimurkar, age 13, shows the creativity of our patients.

Contributors

Matthew J. Hadad, BS
Charles E. Silberstein Research Fellow
Division of Pediatric Orthopaedics
Johns Hopkins Children's Center
Baltimore, Maryland

Paul D. Sponseller, MD, MBA
Sponseller Professor and Head
Division of Pediatric Orthopaedics
Johns Hopkins Medical Institutions
Baltimore, Maryland

1 Anatomy and Normal Development in Children

Paul D. Sponseller

1.1 Introduction

Understanding growth and development is core knowledge in pediatric ortho-paedics. This chapter summarizes clinically relevant anatomy and developmen-tal norms. It also contains a description of normal gait and guidelines for interpreting a gait study.

1.2 Neurodevelopmental Norms

When evaluating a patient at risk of developmental delay, appropriate norms help determine whether a delay is present. This section presents the chrono-logical appearance of key motor, social, and language skills. ▶ Table 1.1 provides the norms for motor milestones.

1.2.1 Psychomotor Skills in Children during Years 1 through 5

- Neonatal period (first month)
  - Supine: Generally flexed and tone a little low.

Table 1.1 Norms for motor milestones

Skill	Mean age (mo)	Std Dev
Roll from back to stomach	3.6	1.4
Roll from stomach to back	4.8	1.4
Sit tailor style	5.3	1.0
Sit unsupported	6.3	1.2
Crawl (many never crawl)	7.8	1.7
Pull to stand	8.1	1.6
Cruise	8.8	1.7
Walk	11.7	2
Run	15	3

Source: Used with permission from Palmer F, Capute A. Keys to developmental assessment. In: McMillan J, ed. Oski's Pediatrics. 3rd ed. Philadelphia, PA: Lippincott Williams & Wilkins; 2006:789.

- 2 Months
  - Prone: Head sustained in plane of body in ventral suspension.
  - Social: Smiles on social contact.
- 4 Months
  - Supine: Reaches and grasps objects and brings them to mouth.
  - Sitting: No head lag on pull to sitting position.
- 4 to 6 Months
  - Prone: Rolls over to supine.
  - Semantics: Turns to his or her own name.
- 6 to 7 Months
  - Sitting: Sits initially with support of pelvis, then independently.
  - Adaptive: Transfers objects from hand to hand.
- 10 Months
  - Standing: Pulls to standing position.
  - Motor: Creeps or crawls.
- 12 to 18 Months
  - Syntax: Speech generally consists of single words).
- 12 Months
  - Motor: Walks with one hand held, "cruises" or walks holding on to furniture.
  - Language: Two "words" besides mama and dada.
- 15 Months
  - Motor: Walks alone, crawls up stairs.
- 18 Months
  - Motor: Runs stiffly.
  - Social: Feeds self.
- 24 Months
  - Motor: Opens doors.
  - Syntax: Uses two- and three-word combinations (telegraphic speech).
- 30 Months
  - Motor: Jumps.
- 36 Months
  - Motor: Goes up stairs alternating feet, stands momentarily on one foot.
- 48 Months
  - Motor: Hops on one foot, throws ball overhand.
- 60 Months
  - Motor: Skips.

1.3 Referral Criteria

Referral to a developmental pediatrician or neurologist should be made if the infant is displaying any of the following:

1. Not rolling by 6 months.
2. Not sitting independently by 8 months.

3. Handedness develops too early (by 12 months): may indicate abnormality of opposite side.
4. Not walking by 18 months.
5. No words by 14 months.

Bibliography

1. Richter SB, Howard BJ, Sturner R. Normal infant and childhood development. In: McMillan J, ed. Oski's Pediatrics. 4th ed. Philadelphia, PA: Lippincott Williams & Wilkins; 2006:593–601
2. WHO Multicentre Growth Reference Study Group. WHO Motor Development Study: windows of achievement for six gross motor development milestones. Acta Paediatr Suppl 2006;450:86–95

1.4 Neurologic Anatomy

1.4.1 Sensation

There is some variation and overlap between levels. This is why injury to a single nerve root may not produce complete loss of sensation within a dermatome. The sensation of proprioception and vibration is carried in the dorsal column of the spinal cord: light touch in the ventral spinothalamic tract and pain and temperature in the lateral spinothalamic tract. During neurologic root recovery, pain sensation returns before light touch (▶ Fig. 1.1).

1.4.2 Upper Extremity Motor Examination

Even though most muscles have innervation from multiple segments, each root has specific muscles and sensory regions for which it is critical. The image shown in ▶ Fig. 1.2 is helpful for diagnosing cervical root lesions and spinal cord injury. Motor testing can be performed in one coordinated sequence, from proximal to distal: deltoid (C5), biceps (C5), wrist extension (C6), finger extension (C7), finger flexion (C8), and finger abduction and adduction (T1).

1.4.3 Upper Extremity Muscle Innervation

Because most muscles are innervated by multiple segments, it is necessary to know all the roots controlling a given muscle. ▶ Fig. 1.3 indicates the roots contributing to a given muscle in the upper extremity. For strength grading, the five-grade scale of the MRC (Medical Research Council) has been widely used:

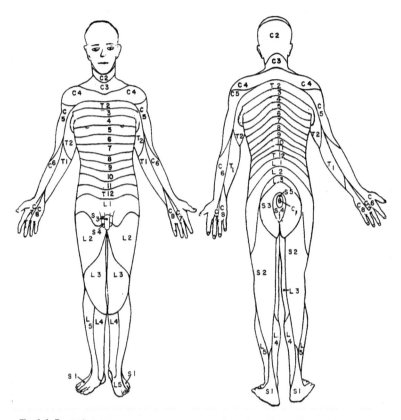

Fig. 1.1 Dermatomes.

- Grade 1: Flicker.
- Grade 2: Less than antigravity.
- Grade 3: Maintains position against gravity.
- Grade 4: Moves against submaximal resistance.
- Grade 5: Full strength.

1.4.4 Formation of the Brachial Plexus

The anatomy is depicted here to understand injuries from birth and later trauma. Most traction injuries involve the upper roots (▶ Fig. 1.4).

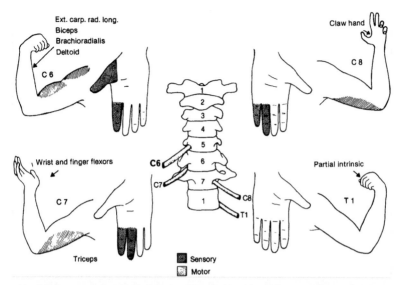

Fig. 1.2 Sensory and motor innervation C6 to T1. Note that only sensory loss is shown in the shaded hand, and only muscle involvement is shown in the arm. (Used with permission from McQueen JD, Khan MI. Neurologic evaluation. In: Sherk HH, Dunn EJ, Eismont FJ, et al, eds. The Cervical Spine. 2nd ed. Philadelphia, PA: J.B. Lippincott; 1989:206 [Figs. 4, 5].)

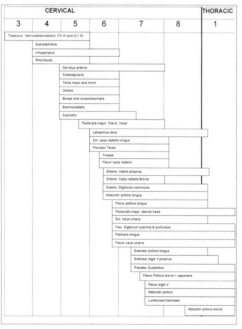

Fig. 1.3 Innervation of muscles of upper extremity.

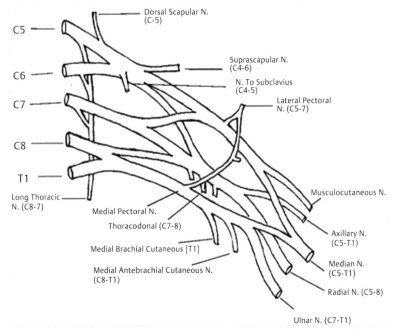

Fig. 1.4 Formation of the brachial plexus.

1.4.5 Peripheral Nerve Testing in the Upper Extremity

The median nerve may be tested by grip or finger flexion and the anterior interosseous nerve (a branch of the median that can be selectively injured) by testing distal interphalangeal flexion of the index finger and thumb, forming an "O."

• Radial nerve: By extending the thumb, the wrist or the metacarpophalangeal joints.
• Ulnar nerve: By crossing fingers, abducting fingers, or flexing the distal interphalangeal joint of the fifth finger (▶ Fig. 1.5).

1.4.6 Lower Extremity Motor Innervation

Knowledge of lower extremity motor innervation is important for understanding spina bifida, lumbar disk herniation, spinal cord injury, and other conditions. Innervation of muscles is by descending spinal segments at progressively

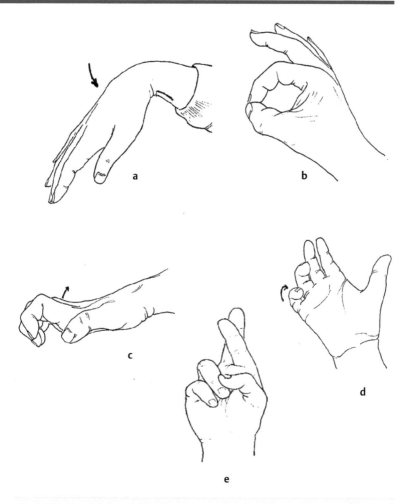

Fig. 1.5 Documentation of the status of all nerves and circulation before treatment of supracondylar humerus fractures. This involves (**a**) checking active palmar flexion (median nerve); (**b**) flexion of distal interphalangeal joints of the index finger and thumb —anterior interosseous nerve; (**c**) dorsiflexion of the metacarpophalangeal joints— posterior interosseous nerve; (**d**) flexion of the fifth finger distal interphalangeal joint; or (**e**) crossing of index and second fingers—ulnar nerve.

distal levels of the limb, with the notable exception of gluteus maximus, medius, and minimus (L5 through S2).

The most important motor innervations to know are iliopsoas (L1 through L3), adductors (L2 through L4), quadriceps (L2 through L4), hamstrings (L4 through L5), anterior tibialis (L4 through L5), gastrocnemius (S1), and glutei (L5 through S2) (▶ Fig. 1.6).

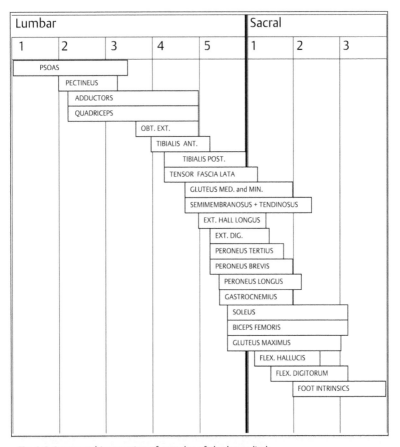

Fig. 1.6 Segmental innervation of muscles of the lower limb.

1.5 Skeletal Development

1.5.1 Appearance of Secondary Ossification Centers and Physeal Closure

In many situations, it is important to know whether an epiphysis should be ossified at a given age, such as in evaluating a patient with a hip dislocation, skeletal dysplasia, or elbow fracture. Normal times for appearance and closure of the long bones are given in ▶ Fig. 1.7; for the hand and foot, see ▶ Fig. 1.8. The following are 11 important milestones:

1. The distal femoral epiphysis is the first to ossify, at ~39 weeks' gestation; the proximal tibia ossifies 1 week later.
2. The mean time for ossification of the proximal femoral epiphysis is 4 months, but normal may be up to 11 months. The greater trochanter ossifies at 4 to 6 years.
3. The triradiate cartilage closes before Risser I.
4. The tarsal navicular does not ossify until 3 to 4 years, so its location must be inferred from the position of the first metatarsal.
5. The last physis to close is that of the medial clavicle, at age 20 to 25 years.

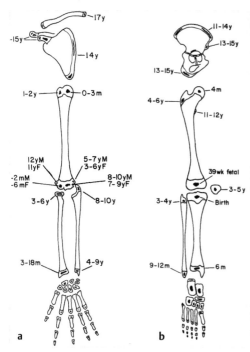

Fig. 1.7 Age of appearance of secondary ossification centers (**a,b**) and physeal closure (*Continued*)

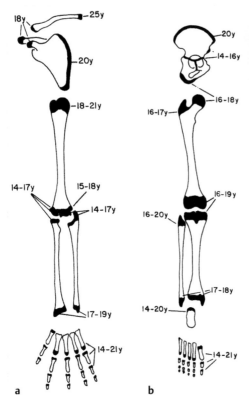

Fig. 1.7 (*Continued*) (**c,d**) in the long bones. (Used with permission from Ogden JA. Radiologic aspects. In: Ogden JA, ed. Skeletal Injury in the Child. 2nd ed. Philadelphia, PA: W.B. Saunders; 1990:84 [Figs. 3-28, 3-29].)

6. The sequence of ossification about the elbow can be remembered by the mnemonic CRITOE (▶ Fig. 1.9):
   a) *C*apitellum (age 2).
   b) *R*adial head (age 5).
   c) *I*nternal epicondyle (age 7).
   d) *T*rochlea (age 9).
   e) *O*lecranon (age 10).
   f) *E*xternal epicondyle (age 11).
7. *Angle of distal humeral articular surface*: This angle is key to understanding any angular change about the elbow. It is best followed by the Baumann angle, between the humeral shaft and the lateral condylar physis (▶ Fig. 1.10). Its normal value is 72 ± 4 degrees. There is no difference between genders or ages from 2 to 13 years.

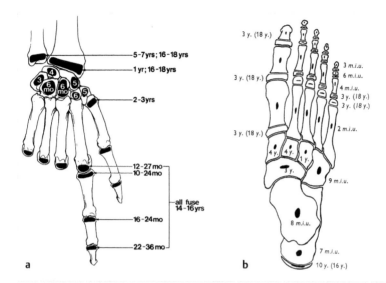

Fig. 1.8 Age of appearance of secondary ossification centers and physeal closure in the hand (**a**) and foot (**b**). m.i.u., months in utero. (**a** is used with permission from O'Brien ET. Fractures of the hand and wrist region. In: Rockwood CA Jr, Wilkins KE, King RE, eds. Fractures in Children. 3rd ed. Philadelphia, PA: J.B. Lippincott Co.; 1991:320 [Fig. 4–1]. **b** is used with permission from Aitken JT, Causey G, Joseph J, Young JZ. The foot. In: Aitken JT, Causey G, Joseph J, Young JZ, eds. A Manual of Human Anatomy: Vol IV, Lower Limb. 2nd ed. Edinburgh: E & S Livingstone; 1966:80 [Fig. 30].)

8. Determination of skeletal age using the elbow: This can be determined by the olecranon or modified Sauvegrain method (▶ Fig. 1.11). The five stages are (1) bipartite olecranon; (2) half-moon–shaped olecranon; (3) rectangular olecranon; (4) partially fused; or (5) fully fused. They occur at 6-month intervals of skeletal age from 11 years in girls and 13 years in boys. The rectangular shape of the olecranon marks the early part of the peak growth velocity. The fully fused olecranon occurs at skeletal age of 13 in girls and 15 in boys, marking the deceleration of growth velocity.
9. Determination of skeletal age using the Sanders Skeletal Maturity Staging System (▶ Table 1.2; ▶ Fig. 1.12). Patients with curves over 30 degrees at stages 3 to 4 are at high risk of progression to surgery, and patients with curves less than 20 degrees at these stages are at low risk.
10. Skeletal age can also be assessed more simply by use of the Thumb Ossification Composite Index or TOCI (▶ Fig. 1.13).

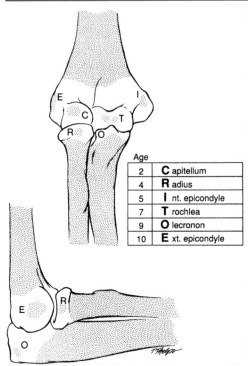

Fig. 1.9 Appearance of age of ossification centers about the elbow can be summarized by the mnemonic "CRITOE." (Used with permission from Sponseller PD. Orthopaedic injuries. In: Nichols DG, Yaster M, Lappe DG, Buck JR, eds. Golden Hour: The Handbook of Advanced Pediatric Life Support. St. Louis, MO: Mosby Year Book; 1991:350 [Fig. 18–3].)

Age	
2	**C** apitellum
4	**R** adius
5	**I** nt. epicondyle
7	**T** rochlea
9	**O** lecronon
10	**E** xt. epicondyle

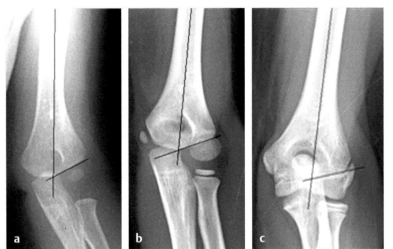

Fig. 1.10 (a–c) Differing configuration of the distal humerus and landmarks used for measurement of the Baumann angle.

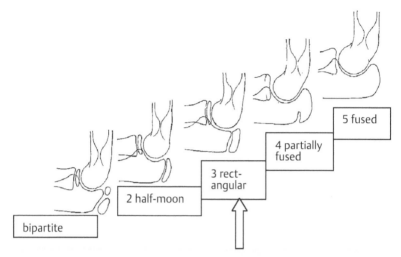

Fig. 1.11 Simplified Sauvegrain method for skeletal maturity assessment.

11. Determination of skeletal maturity using the calcaneal apophysis: this occurs in six stages, four of them prior to peak height velocity (PHV). Thus, it is ideal for predicting the PHV, which occurs between stages 3 and 4. Stage 2 occurs about 2 years before PHV, stage 3 about 1 year prior, and stage 4 just after (▶ Fig. 1.14).

Bibliography

1. Nicholson AD, Liu RW, Sanders JO, Cooperman DR. Relationship of calcaneal and iliac apophyseal ossification to peak height velocity timing in children. J Bone Joint Surg Am 2015;97(2):147–154

1.5.2 Cervical Spine Radiographic Normal Values for Children

Alignment

1. The cervical spine in children is characterized by increased mobility at C2–C3, termed *pseudosubluxation*, which should not exceed 3 mm.
2. The tip of the odontoid should not be more than 1 cm from the basion of the skull (anterior rim of the foramen magnum).

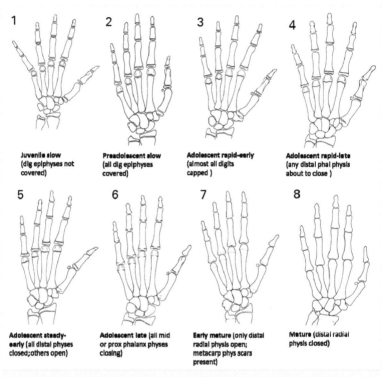

1 Juvenile slow (dig epiphyses not covered)

2 Preadolescent slow (all dig epiphyses covered)

3 Adolescent rapid–early (almost all digits capped)

4 Adolescent rapid–late (any distal phal physis about to close)

5 Adolescent steady-early (all distal physes closed;others open)

6 Adolescent late (all mid or prox phalanx physes closing)

7 Early mature (only distal radial physis open; metacarp phys scars present)

8 Mature (distal radial physis closed)

Fig. 1.12 Simplified Tanner-Whitehouse III (Sanders) maturation scale for skeletal maturity assessment. Note that the distal phalangeal epiphyses are the key to the curve acceleration phase (CAP). When they are capped, the phase is beginning, and when they are all closed, the phase has ended. Stage 1: All digital epiphyses not covered (epiphyses not as wide as metaphyses). Stage 2: All digital epiphyses are covered. Stage 3: Most epiphyses cap their metaphyses. Capping is a small bend over the metaphyseal edge. This is also the beginning of the CAP. Stage 4: At least one of distal phalanges closed. Stages 5 to 8: Descending phases of growth. (Adapted with permission from Sanders JO, Khoury JG, Kishan S, et al. Predicting scoliosis progression from skeletal maturity: a simplified classification during adolescence. J Bone Joint Surg Am. 2008;90(3):540–553.)

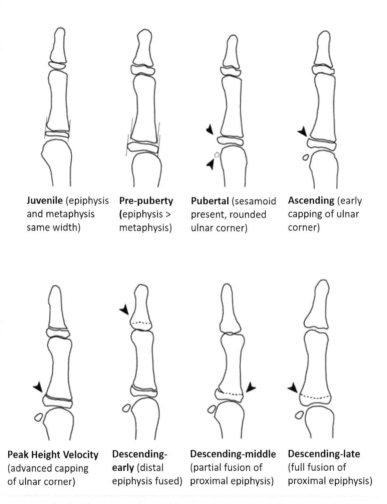

Juvenile (epiphysis and metaphysis same width)

Pre-puberty (epiphysis > metaphysis)

Pubertal (sesamoid present, rounded ulnar corner)

Ascending (early capping of ulnar corner)

Peak Height Velocity (advanced capping of ulnar corner)

Descending-early (distal epiphysis fused)

Descending-middle (partial fusion of proximal epiphysis)

Descending-late (full fusion of proximal epiphysis)

Fig. 1.13 The thumb axis provides similar information to the whole hand. Thumb Ossification Composite Index (TOCI) stages 1 through 8 are based on the appearance of the ulnar sesamoid and the maturation of the phalangeal physes. Peak height velocity occurs between TOCI stages 4 and 5, and menarche occurs in TOCI stage 6. TOCI stage 8 matches Sanders 7, with less than 1–2 cm growth remaining.

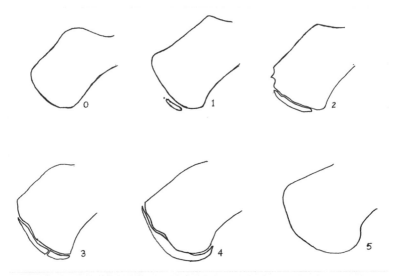

Fig. 1.14 Determination of skeletal maturity using the calcaneal apophysis:
Stage 0: no apophysis.
Stage 1: <50% coverage.
Stage 2: >50% coverage.
Stage 3: Complete coverage within 2 mm of plantar edge. ~1 year before peak height velocity (PHV).
Stage 4: Beginning fusion; just after PHV.
Stage 5: Complete fusion.

Table 1.2 Key findings of the simplified Tanner–Whitehouse III skeletal maturity assessment

Stage	Key features	Tanner–Whitehouse III stage	Greulich and Pyle reference	Related maturity signs
1. Juvenile slow	Digital epiphyses not covered	Some digits are at stage E or lower	Female 8 y + 10 mo, male 12 y + 6 mo (note fifth middle phalanx)	Tanner stage 1
2. Preadolescent slow	All digital epiphyses covered	All digits at stage F	Female 10 y, male 13 y	Tanner stage 2, starting growth spurt

Table 1.2 (*continued*)

Stage	Key features	Tanner–Whitehouse III stage	Greulich and Pyle reference	Related maturity signs
3. Adolescent rapid-early	Preponderance of digits is capped. The 2nd through 5th metacarpal epiphyses wider than their metaphyses	All digits are at stage G	Female 11 and 12 y, male 13 y + 6 mo and 14 y	Peak height velocity, Risser stage 0, open pelvic triradiate cartilage
4. Adolescent rapid-late	Any distal phalangeal physes are clearly beginning to close	Any distal phalanges are at stage H	Female 13 y (digits 2, 3, 4), male 15 y (digits 4, 5)	Girls typically in Tanner stage 3, Risser stage 0, open triradiate cartilage
5. Adolescent steady-early	All distal phalangeal physes closed; others are open	All distal phalanges and thumb metacarpal are at stage I; others remain at stage G	Female 13 y + 6 mo, male 15 y + 6 mo	Risser stage 0, triradiate cartilage closed, menarche only; occasionally starts earlier
6. Adolescent steady-late	Middle or proximal phalangeal physes are closing	Middle or proximal phalanges are at stages H and I	Female 14 y, male 16 y (late)	Risser sign positive (stage 1 or more)
7. Early mature	Only distal radial physis is open; metacarpal physeal scars may be present	All digits are at stage I. The distal radial physis is at stage G or H	Female 15 y, male 17 y	Risser stage 4
8. Mature	Distal radial physis completely closed	All digits are at stage I	Female 17 y, male 19 y	Risser stage 5

Source: Used with permission from Sanders JO, Khoury JG, Kishan S, et al. Predicting scoliosis progression from skeletal maturity: a simplified classification during adolescence. J Bone Joint Surg Am 2008;90(3):541 (Table 1).

3. The physis of the odontoid normally fuses between 3 and 6 years.
4. The atlas–dens interval should be less than 4 mm.
5. The power ratio is the ratio of the distance from basion to the posterior arch of C1 divided by the distance from the opisthion to the anterior arch of C1. This ratio should be less than 1.
6. The retropharyngeal space should not exceed 8 mm; if greater, it could signify bleeding from a fracture or a dislocation.
7. The spinal laminae should form a smooth line posteriorly.
8. The vertebral bodies may be wedged anteriorly, especially on their superior surfaces, until age 10 years (▶ Fig. 1.15).

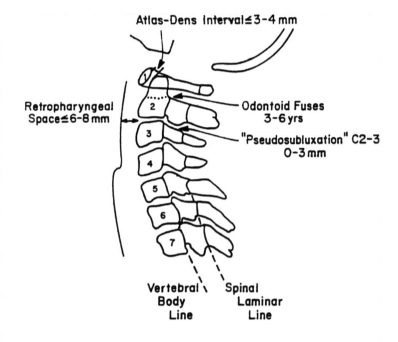

These values are valid until the age of 10.

Fig. 1.15 Normal values of cervical spine alignment for children. (Used with permission from Sponseller PD. Orthopaedic injuries. In: Nichols DG, Yaster M, Lappe DG, Buck JR, eds. Golden Hour: The Handbook of Advanced Pediatric Life Support. St. Louis, MO: Mosby Year Book; 1991:353 [Fig. 18–4].)

1.5.3 Development of the Cervical Spine

First Cervical Vertebra (Atlas)

1. Body: Not ossified at birth; the center (occasionally two centers) appears during the first year after birth.
2. Neural arches: Appear bilaterally at approximately the seventh fetal week; most of the anterior portion of the superior articulating surface is usually formed by the body.
3. Synchondrosis of posterior arch: Unites by the third year. Union rarely is preceded by the appearance of a secondary center within the synchondrosis.
4. Neurocentral synchondrosis: Fuses at approximately the seventh year (▶ Fig. 1.16).

Second Cervical Vertebra (Axis)

1. Body: One center (occasionally two) appears by the fifth fetal month.
2. Neural arches: Appear bilaterally by fetal month 7.
3. Neural arches fuse posteriorly by year 2 or 3.
4. Bifid tip of spinous process: Occasionally a secondary center is present in each tip.
5. Neurocentral synchondrosis: Fuses at 3 to 6 years.
6. Inferior epiphyseal ring: Appears at puberty and fuses at around 25 years.
7. "Summit" ossification center for odontoid: Appears at 3 to 6 years and fuses with the odontoid by 12 years.
8. Odontoid (dens). Two separate centers appear by fetal month 5 and fuse with each other by month 7.

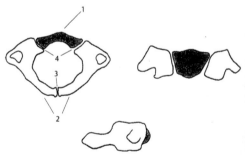

Fig. 1.16 Axial, coronal, and sagittal views of the developing atlas. The first cervical vertebra is formed by three ossification sites: the anterior arch (*gray*), or centrum, and the two neural arches (*white*). (Used with permission from Oh BC, Wang MY. Cervical anatomy and surgical approaches. In: Kim DH, Betz RR, Huhn SL, Newton PO, eds. Surgery of the Pediatric Spine. New York: Thieme; 2008:95 [Fig. 8–1].)

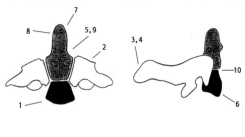

Fig. 1.17 Coronal and sagittal views of the developing axis. There are four ossification centers present at birth: one center for each neural arch (*white*), one for the odontoid process (*gray*), and one for the body (*black*). (Used with permission from Oh BC, Wang MY. Cervical anatomy and surgical approaches. In: Kim DH, Betz RR, Huhn SL, Newton PO. Surgery of the Pediatric Spine. New York: Thieme; 2008:96 [Fig. 8–2].)

9. Synchondrosis between odontoid and neural arch: Fuses at 3 to 6 years.
10. Synchondrosis between odontoid and body: Fuses at 3 to 6 years (▶ Fig. 1.17).

1.5.4 Spinal Growth

The growth of the spine occurs relatively earlier than that of the extremities, but after the extreme of cranial growth. If arthrodesis is considered in a growing child, the following rules will help predict the consequences for growth.

Guidelines and Rules of Thumb

1. T1–S1 growth rates:
   a) 0 to 5 years: 2 cm/year.
   b) 6 to 10 years: 0.9 cm/year.
   c) 10 + years: 1.8 cm/year through growth spurt.
2. Growth of the T1–S1 segment is two-thirds complete by 6 years.
3. Growth remaining from T1–S1 at age 5 is 15 cm.
4. DiMeglio has summarized the growth of the extremities and spine with respect to maturity indicators (elbow growth centers, Risser sign, menarche, triradiate cartilage closure) in ▶ Fig. 1.18. Triradiate cartilage closure slightly precedes the peak height velocity, olecranon closure occurs at the peak height velocity, and menarche occurs just after peak height velocity; all occur at or before Risser sign turns to 1.

Note that posterior arthrodesis alone does not stop growth completely within a fused segment. Further growth can cause relative compression of disk space, exacerbation of preexisting lordosis, or rotation of scoliosis ("crankshaft"; ▶ Fig. 1.19).

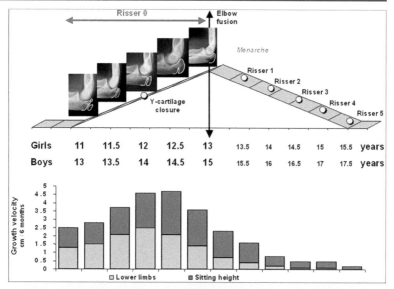

Fig. 1.18 Simplified skeletal age assessment with the olecranon method during the accelerating pubertal growth phase of peak height velocity and Risser grade 0 from the ages of 11 to 13 years in boys, with a decelerating growth phase after elbow fusion. Y cartilage closure = triradiate cartilage closure. (Used with permission from Charles YP, Dimeglio A, Canavese F, Daures JP. Skeletal age assessment from the olecranon for idiopathic scoliosis at Risser grade 0. J Bone Joint Surg Am 2007:89(12):2739 [Fig. 1].)

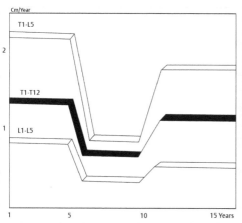

Fig. 1.19 Approximate growth velocity of the spine by segments: thoracic, lumbar, and combined segments. Note that the greatest velocity is in preschool years, and then a significant drop occurs. (Used with permission from Dimeglio A. Growth of the spine before age 5 years. J Pediatr Orthop B 1992;1(2):103 [Fig. 7].)

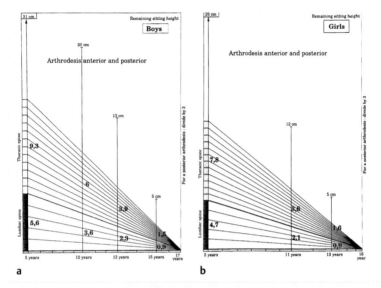

Fig. 1.20 Growth remaining in the spine by segment for (**a**) boys and (**b**) girls. Note that the remaining component of sitting height is due to the head, cervical spine, and cranium. (Used with permission from Dimeglio A. Growth of the spine before age 5 years. J Pediatr Orthop B 1992;1(2):104 [Figs. 11 and 12].)

Spinal Growth Remaining Calculation

• 0.07 cm × number of spinal segments × growth years left (▶ Fig. 1.20).

1.5.5 Extremity Growth: Relative Contributions to Growth of the Long Bones

The contributions of each physis to longitudinal growth are a reflection of its activity, which in turn influences remodeling potential. A simple rule of thumb is that most growth occurs "away from the elbow and at the knee" in the upper and lower extremities, respectively (▶ Fig. 1.21).

Some guidelines for estimating growth:
1. At each physis, this estimation can be done during the preadolescent years using the approximate rates:
   a) Proximal femur: ⅛ inch/year.
   b) Distal femur: ⅜ inch/year.
   c) Proximal tibia: ¼ inch/year.
   d) Distal tibia: 3/16 inch/year.

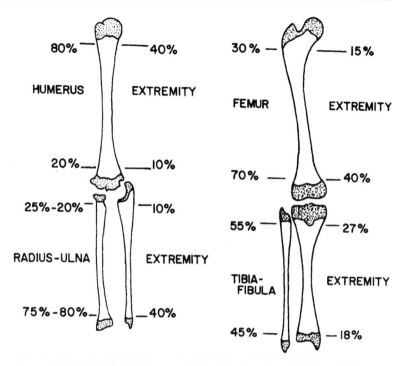

Fig. 1.21 Relative contributions to growth of the long bones of the upper (left) and lower (right) extremity. (Used with permission from Ogden JA. Radiologic aspects. In: Ogden JA, ed. Skeletal Injury in the Child. 2nd ed. Philadelphia, PA: W.B. Saunders; 1990:85 [Fig. 3–30A,B].)

These estimates are true until age 13 for girls or age 15 for boys. For taller-than-average children, these rates are greater. For long growth periods of more than 3 years, it is better to consult growth tables (▶ Fig. 1.22).

1. Total adult height = 2 × height at age 2.
2. Total adult length of lower extremities = 2 × length at age 4.
3. Growth ceases in girls at 15 to 15.5 years, in boys at 17 to 17.5 years.
4. Another way to estimate adult height:
   a) Males = (father's height + mother's height + 6 cm)/2.
   b) Females = (father's height + mother's height – 6 cm)/2.
   c) Two standard deviations = ±5 cm.
5. Another method to estimate adult height is to use the multiplier method (▶ Table 1.3). This takes into account the fact that existing height is a strong predictor of final height.

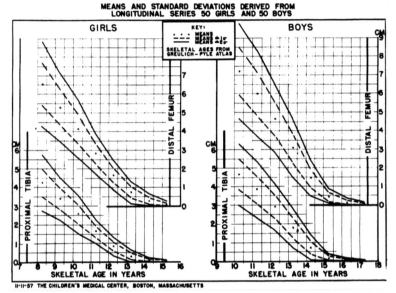

GROWTH REMAINING IN NORMAL DISTAL FEMUR AND PROXIMAL TIBIA FOLLOWING CONSECUTIVE SKELETAL AGE LEVELS

MEANS AND STANDARD DEVIATIONS DERIVED FROM
LONGITUDINAL SERIES 50 GIRLS AND 50 BOYS

Fig. 1.22 Growth remaining in normal distal femur and proximal tibia following consecutive skeletal ages. (Used with permission from Anderson M, Green WT, Messner MB. Growth and predictions of growth in the lower extremities. J Bone Joint Surg Am 1963;45(1):10 [Chart III].)

Table 1.3 Multiplier method for height (the Paley method)[a]

Age (y)	Height multiplier	
	Girls	Boys
Birth	3.30	3.53
0.5	2.50	2.64
1.0	2.22	2.34
1.5	2.04	2.16
2.0	1.92	2.04
2.5	1.81	1.94
3.0	1.73	1.86
3.5	1.68	1.78
4.0	1.62	1.73

Table 1.3 (*continued*)

Age (y)	Height multiplier	
	Girls	Boys
4.5	1.57	1.67
5.0	1.51	1.63
5.5	1.47	1.58
6.0	1.42	1.53
6.5	1.38	1.50
7.0	1.34	1.45
7.5	1.31	1.42
8.0	1.28	1.38
8.5	1.25	1.35
9.0	1.23	1.32
9.5	1.21	1.30
10.0	1.18	1.28
10.5	1.16	1.26
11.0	1.13	1.23
11.5	1.11	1.21
12.0	1.08	1.19
12.5	1.06	1.16
13.0	1.04	1.13
13.5	1.03	1.11
14.0	1.02	1.08
14.5	1.01	1.06
15.0	1.01	1.04
15.5	1.01	1.03
16.0	1.00	1.02
16.5	1.00	1.01
17.0	1.00	1.01
17.5	1.00	1.01
18.0	1.00	1.00

[a]The patient's existing height may be multiplied by a number on this table corresponding to age to determine final height.

Growth Curves for Long Bones

Growth curves are useful when absolute lengths are needed. ▶ Fig. 1.23 and ▶ Fig. 1.24 represent the same population data as presented differently in the "growth remaining" curves.

Growth Remaining Curves

These are a reformulation of the data shown in ▶ Fig. 1.23 and ▶ Fig. 1.24. This format is especially useful for estimating the effects of physeal closure. One must know the patient's skeletal age and percentile rank for height.

Longitudinal Growth from Distal Tibial and Fibular Physes

1. Distal tibial and fibular physeal fractures often occur in childhood and adolescence. Growth plate damage may occur. Physeal closure in either bone then must be evaluated for significance of both shortening and angular deformity.

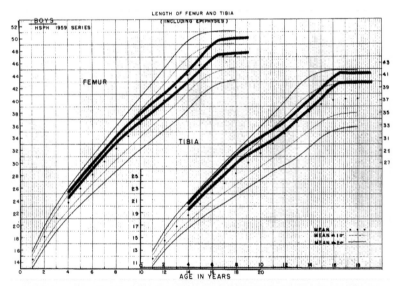

Fig. 1.23 Length of normal femur and tibia for boys (including epiphyses). (Used with permission from Anderson M, Messner MB, Green WT. Distribution of lengths of the normal femur and tibia in children from one to eighteen years of age. J Bone Joint Surg Am 1964;46(6):1201 [Chart II].)

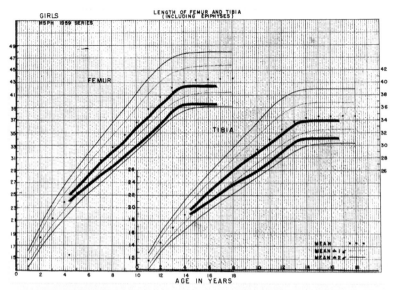

Fig. 1.24 Length of normal femur and tibia for girls (including epiphyses). (Used with permission from Anderson M, Messner MB, Green WT. Distribution of lengths of the normal femur and tibia in children from one to eighteen years of age. J Bone Joint Surg Am 1964;46(6):1200 [Chart I].)

2. The following growth-remaining graphs may be used for prediction of the deformity. The percentile to follow for a given patient may be obtained from the percentile of the patient's rank in ▶ Fig. 1.23, ▶ Fig. 1.24, and ▶ Fig. 1.25.
3. Length lost from total arrest may be calculated. In general, inequality of less than 1 cm is of no clinical significance.
4. Prediction of angular growth disturbance as a result of peripheral arrest may be calculated from the growth remaining and the width of the physis. Because the average distal tibia is 4 to 5 cm wide, 10 degrees of angulation is likely to occur in boys with a peripheral growth arrest before the age of 13½ and in girls before 11½.
5. This may also be used to predict the effects of surgical hemiepiphysiodesis.

Straight-Line Graph for Predictions of Discrepancy

For growth disturbances that do not change characteristics over time, if skeletal age is known, the eventual inequality of limb length at maturity can be calculated by plotting data points on the straight-line graph developed by Moseley (▶ Fig. 1.26; ▶ Fig. 1.27). The procedure is explained step by step. Conditions

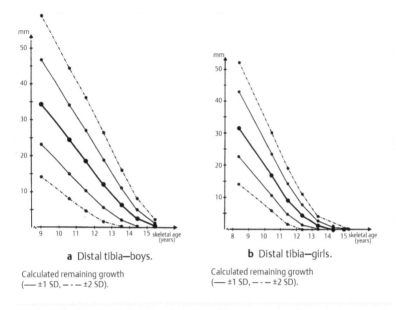

a Distal tibia—boys.

Calculated remaining growth
(—— ±1 SD, — - — ±2 SD).

b Distal tibia—girls.

Calculated remaining growth
(—— ±1 SD, — - — ±2 SD).

Fig. 1.25 Growth remaining in distal tibia (mean ± 2 SD) for boys (**a**) and girls (**b**). (Used with permission from Karrholm J, Hansson LI, Selvik G. Longitudinal growth rate of the distal tibia and fibula in children. Clin Orthop Relat Res 1984;191:124 [Figs. 2B and 3B].)

for which the graph may not be appropriate are those with a phasic nature, for example, a discrepancy that is due to juvenile rheumatoid arthritis or Klippel–Trenaunay syndrome.

Upper Extremity Growth

Growth arrest occurs less commonly in the upper extremity. Occasionally, however, as a result of infection, tumor, or trauma, growth is affected, and it may become necessary to calculate the resulting discrepancy (▶ Fig. 1.28).

Overall Physical Growth Norms

Physical growth norms include mean stature for age and their respective percentiles. They are useful in screening for growth disturbances and estimating height at maturity (▶ Fig. 1.29; ▶ Fig. 1.30).

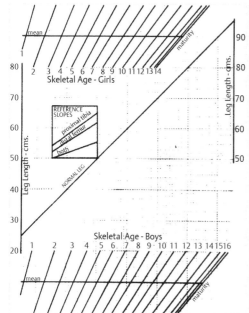

Fig. 1.26 Moseley straight-line graph for predicting limb-length inequality. (Used with permission from Moseley CF. A straight-line graph for leg-length discrepancies. J Bone Joint Surg Am 1977;59(2):176 [Fig. 1].)

1.5.6 The Multiplier Method for Growth Prediction

The multiplier method can be used to predict the growth of long bones or the entire stature so long as the growth is occurring naturally without any intervention. It uses the patient's own initial growth data and multiplies that by a figure known to be the proportion of growth remaining. Therefore, the growth of one limb or one bone can be calculated from just one measurement. If a growing patient has a limb-length discrepancy, then that discrepancy is multiplied by the multiplier to calculate the final discrepancy. ► Table 1.3 and ► Table 1.4 present the multipliers for different ages.

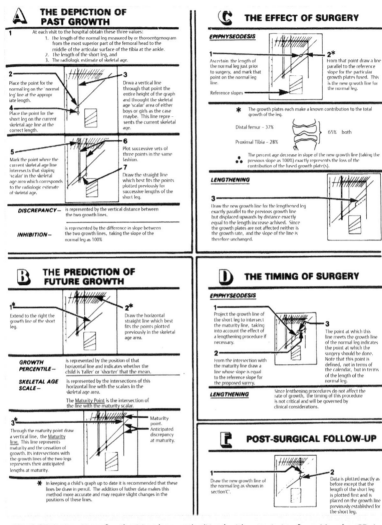

Fig. 1.27 Instructions for the Moseley graph. (Used with permission from Moseley CF. A straight-line graph for leg-length discrepancies. J Bone Joint Surg Am 1977;59(2):177 [Fig. 2].)

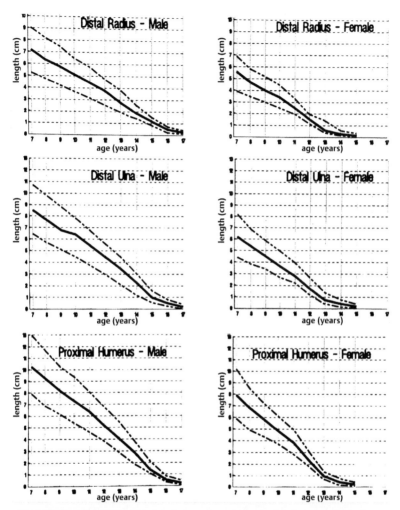

Fig. 1.28 Growth remaining from major upper extremity physes. These graphs are from the Child Research Counsel, Denver, Colorado. Mean (*solid line*) and two standard deviations (*dotted lines*). (Used with permission from Bortel DT, Pritchett JW. Straight-line graphs for the prediction of growth of the upper extremities. J Bone Joint Surg Am 1993;75(6):889 [Fig. 2].)

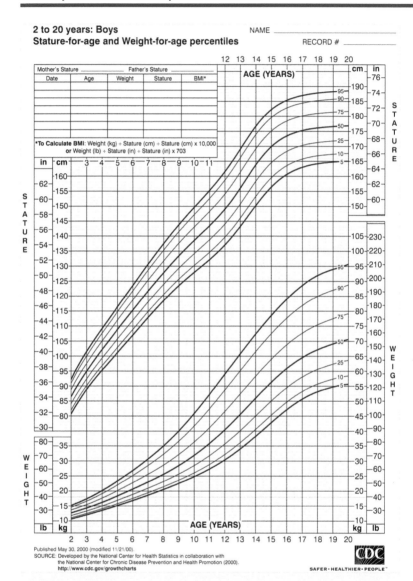

Fig. 1.29 Age 2 to 20 years for boys: stature-for-age and weight-for-age percentiles.

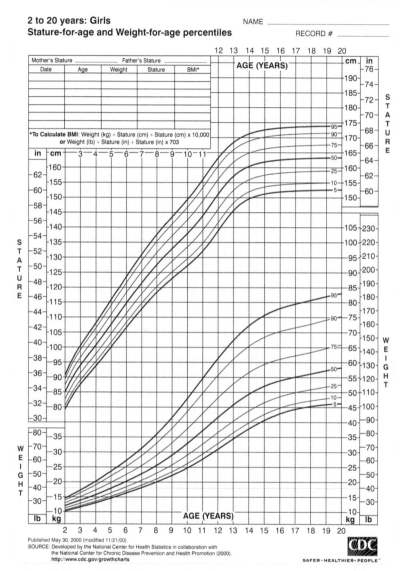

Fig. 1.30 Age 2 to 20 years for girls: stature-for-age and weight-for-age percentiles.

Table 1.4 Multiplier method for lower limb lengths[a]

Age (y + mo)	Lower limb length multiplier	
	Girls	Boys
Birth	4.630	5.080
0 + 3	4.155	4.550
0 + 6	3.725	4.050
0 + 9	3.300	3.600
1 + 0	2.970	3.240
1 + 3	2.750	2.975
1 + 6	2.600	2.825
1 + 9	2.490	2.700
2 + 0	2.390	2.590
2 + 3	2.295	2.480
2 + 6	2.200	2.385
2 + 9	2.125	2.300
3 + 0	2.050	2.230
3 + 6	1.925	2.110
4 + 0	1.830	2.000
4 + 6	1.740	1.890
5 + 0	1.660	1.820
5 + 6	1.580	1.740
6 + 0	1.510	1.670
6 + 6	1.460	1.620
7 + 0	1.430	1.570
7 + 6	1.370	1.520
8 + 0	1.330	1.470
8 + 6	1.290	1.420
9 + 0	1.260	1.380
9 + 6	1.220	1.340
10 + 0	1.190	1.310
10 + 6	1.160	1.280
11 + 0	1.130	1.240
11 + 6	1.100	1.220
12 + 0	1.070	1.180
12 + 6	1.050	1.160
13 + 0	1.030	1.130
13 + 6	1.010	1.100

Table 1.4 (continued)

Age (y + mo)	Lower limb length multiplier	
	Girls	Boys
14 + 0	1.000	1.080
14 + 6	NA	1.060
15 + 0	NA	1.040
15 + 6	NA	1.020
16 + 0	NA	1.010
16 + 6	NA	1.010
17 + 0	NA	1.000

Abbreviation: NA, not applicable.
Source: Used with permission from Paley D, Bhave A, Herzenberg JE, Bowen JR. Multiplier method for predicting limb-length discrepancy. J Bone Joint Surg Am 2000;82(10):1440 (Table 5).
[a]The patient's limb-length inequality may be multiplied by a number from this table corresponding to age to determine the final discrepancy. It may also be used to calculate the amount of growth remaining in the lower limb.

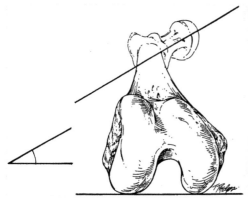

Fig. 1.31 Femoral anteversion: definition.

1.5.7 Alignment in the Transverse Plane

1. *Femoral anteversion* is the angle between the plane of the femoral head and neck and that of the posterior surface of the femoral condyles (▶ Fig. 1.31). Femoral anteversion declines steadily in normal children from a mean of 25 degrees at birth to 15 degrees at adulthood (▶ Fig. 1.32). It may be followed clinically by recording internal and external rotation of the hip in extension. It can be estimated in the clinic with the patient prone by internally rotating

35

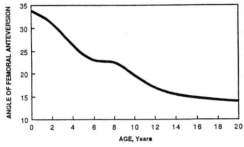

Fig. 1.32 Normal values for femoral anteversion. (Used with permission from Shands AR Jr, Steele MK. Torsion of the femur. J Bone Joint Surg Am 1958;40(4):806 [Graph I].)

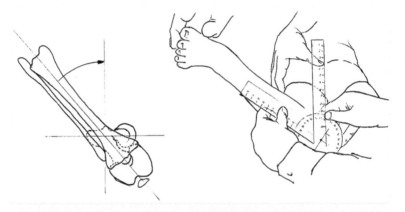

Fig. 1.33 Clinical measurement of femoral anteversion. This may be estimated with the patient prone by rotating the hip internally until the greater trochanter has reached maximal prominence and then noting the angle formed by the tibia with a vertical line.

the hip until the greater trochanter is considered to be directly lateral and measuring the angle formed by the flexed tibia with the vertical (▶ Fig. 1.33). Anteversion is most accurately measured by computed tomography (CT) (▶ Fig. 1.34). Anteversion can also be measured by standard radiographs using techniques of Ogata or Magilligan.

2. CT measurement of anteversion: On sequential cuts by CT, a line is drawn through the centers of the femoral head and base of the neck. Another line is drawn through the posterior surfaces of the femoral condyles. The angle between these two lines is the femoral anteversion (▶ Fig. 1.34).

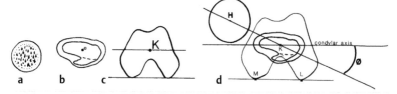

Fig. 1.34 Measurement of anteversion by computed tomography. (**a**) Center of femoral head. (**b**) Center of base of femoral neck. (**c**) Condylar axis. (**d**) Anteversion is the angle between the two lines so defined. If the femoral head is posterior to the condylar axis, the value of the angle is negative and is termed retroversion. H, hip; K, knee; L, lateral; M, medial. (Used with permission from Murphy SB, Simon SR, Kijewski PK, Wilkinson RH, Griscom NT. Femoral anteversion. J Bone Joint Surg Am 1987;69(8):1175 [Fig. 10].).

Bibliography

1. Magilligan DJ. Calculation of the angle of anteversion by means of horizontal lateral roentgenography. J Bone Joint Surg Am 1956;38-A(6):1231–1246
2. Murphy SB, Simon SR, Kijewski PK, Wilkinson RH, Griscom NT. Femoral anteversion. J Bone Joint Surg Am 1987;69(8):1169–1176

3. Ogata method of determining femoral anteversion using biplane radiographs:
   a) This method can be used when CT is not readily available. It uses graphs to provide trigonometric calculations of anteversion as well as true neck–shaft angle from two standardized plain radiographs (▶ Fig. 1.35; ▶ Fig. 1.36). It is based on the fact that the tibia is perpendicular to the condylar axis when the knee is flexed. The method is accurate when positioning is done carefully, within ± 6 degrees for anteversion and ± 5 degrees for true neck–shaft angle.
   b) Technique for obtaining radiographs: The patient is positioned with the knee flexed 90 degrees and perpendicular to the surface of the radiography table. This places the condylar plane of the femur in a true horizontal position. A projected anteroposterior neck–shaft radiograph is taken, and the angle is drawn and labeled α. The patient is then positioned on the side, with the knee flexed and the tibia horizontal. A projected lateral neck–shaft radiograph is taken, and the angle is drawn and labeled β.
   c) Using the graphs in ▶ Fig. 1.37 and ▶ Fig. 1.38, values for true neck–shaft angle and anteversion can be obtained.

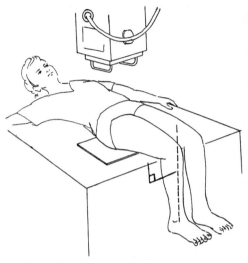

Fig. 1.35 Positioning for the "projected AP femur X-ray" in the method of Ogata. The projected neck–shaft angle obtained from this film is labeled α and used in the next step in Fig. 1.37 and Fig. 1.38.

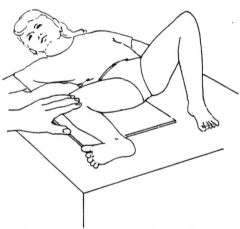

Fig. 1.36 Positioning for the "projected lateral femur X-ray" in the method of Ogata. The tibia should be freely resting flat on the cassette. The projected neck–shaft angle obtained from this film is labeled β and is used in the next step in ▶ Fig. 1.37 and ▶ Fig. 1.38.

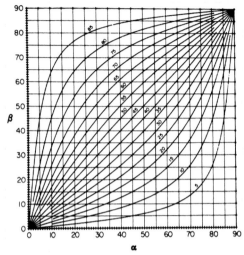

Fig. 1.37 Determination of true anteversion of the femur using the intersection of projected anteroposterior (α) and lateral (β). (Used with permission from Ogata K, Goldsand EM. A simple biplanar method of measuring femoral anteversion and neck-shaft angle. J Bone Joint Surg Am 1979;61 (6):849 [Fig. 5A].)

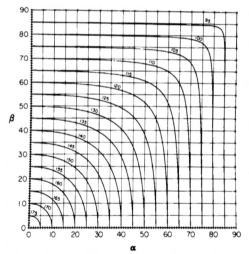

Fig. 1.38 Determination of true neck-shaft angle. (Used with permission from Ogata K, Goldsand EM. A simple biplanar method of measuring femoral anteversion and neck-shaft angle. J Bone Joint Surg Am 1979;61(6):849 [Fig. 5B].)

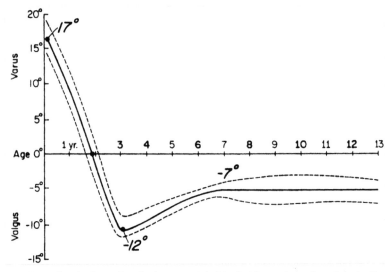

Fig. 1.39 The tibiofemoral angle during growth. (Used with permission from Salenius P, Vankka E. The development of the tibiofemoral angle in children. J Bone Joint Surg Am 1975;57(2):260 [Fig. 1].)

1.5.8 Development of the Tibiofemoral Angle during Growth

The coronal tibiofemoral angle changes dramatically during the first 5 years of life—from varus to excessive valgus to "normal" valgus. This was illustrated by Salenius in the graph redrawn in ▶ Fig. 1.39. It was made from clinical measurements on 1,000 normal children. Radiographs are not generally clinically necessary in the first 12 to 18 months of life. Chapters 2, 3, and 4 of this book detail the interpretation of abnormal conditions.

Alignment of the Lower Extremity

1. Knowledge of normal tibiofemoral alignment is essential for planning osteotomies around the knee. Normal values vary slightly, depending on the width of the pelvis and limb lengths.
2. Definitions:
   a) *Mechanical axis* is the angle of two lines between the centers of the hip, knee, and ankle; normal angle is 0 degrees, inclined 3 degrees from the vertical.

b) *Anatomic axis* is the angle between the tibial and femoral diaphyses; normal is 6 degrees.
c) The knee joint line should be horizontal.
d) Femoral joint angle is 90 − (β + Θ).
e) Tibial joint angle is 90 − Θ (▶ Fig. 1.40).

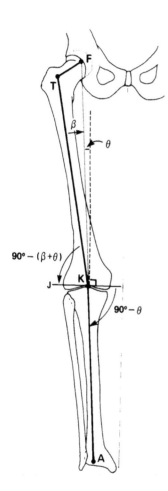

Fig. 1.40 Alignment of lower extremity. In normal subjects, β = 6 degrees and Θ = 3 degrees, but these may vary depending on the distance between the hip centers, femoral neck–shaft angle, and limb length A, ankle; F, femoral; K, knee; T, trochanter base.

1.5.9 Clinical Evaluation of Rotation of the Lower Extremities

Rotational abnormalities can be approached in a systematic fashion. Foot progression angle quantifies the sum of rotations occurring in the femur, tibia, and foot. These components may be assessed by the parameters pictured on the following pages. Normal ranges throughout growth for all of these parameters are given, as determined by Staheli et al. Treatment for these rotational deformities is rarely indicated, but showing the natural progression to the parents in graphic form can be helpful.

Metatarsal adduction and abduction (▶ Fig. 1.41; ▶ Fig. 1.42): Forefoot adduction is generally recorded from clinical measurements. Metatarsal adduction can be quantified by drawing a line through the heel bisector and noting which toe it intersects. Normally, it falls between the second and third toes. Moderate to severe adduction is present when the line falls lateral to the fourth toe.

The foot progression angle is the end product of all rotational components in the lower extremity: hip, femur, knee, tibia, and foot. It is the angle formed by the foot (on the average) with the direction of walking (▶ Fig. 1.43).

The *thigh–foot angle* is an approximate clinical measure of tibial torsion. It is assessed with the patient prone and the ankle gently dorsiflexed to a neutral position (▶ Fig. 1.44a). Normal values with age are given in ▶ Fig. 1.44b. When the foot is unable to provide a satisfactory reference because of a rotational problem, such as clubfoot, metatarsus adductus, spasticity, or contracture, the tibial torsion can be estimated by the *transmalleolar axis*. This is the angle formed by a line between the two malleoli and a line in the middle of the thigh when the patient is prone with the knee bent (▶ Fig. 1.44c).

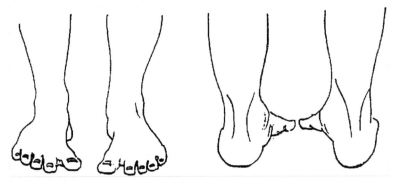

Fig. 1.41 Appearance of metatarsus adductus.

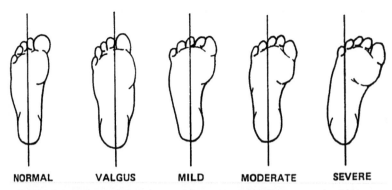

NORMAL   **VALGUS**   **MILD**   **MODERATE**   **SEVERE**

Fig. 1.42 Quantification of metatarsus adductus. This is done with the child prone. A line is drawn through the middle of the heel and the examiner notes which toe it intersects. (Used with permission from Bleck EE. Developmental orthopaedics. III: Toddlers. Dev Med Child Neurol 1982;24(5):545 [Fig. 20].)

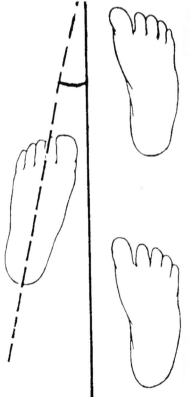

Fig. 1.43 Measurement of the foot progression angle.

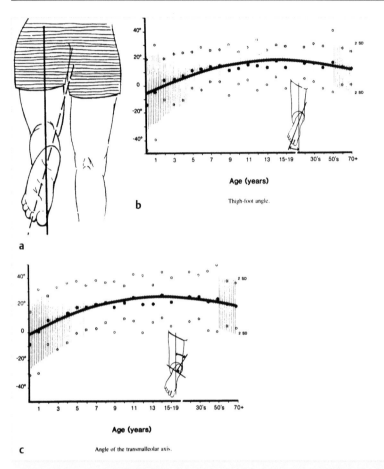

Fig. 1.44 Measurement of the thigh–foot angle. (**a**) Clinical measurement. (**b**) Normal values with age. (**c**) Transmalleolar axis and normal values for age. (**b** and **c** are used with permission from Staheli LT, Corbett M, Wyss C, King H. Lower-extremity rotational problems in children. J Bone Joint Surg Am 1985;67(1):43 [Figs. 2E, 2F].)

Internal and external rotations of the hip in extension are used to assess the relative contributions of the hip to rotation (▶ Fig. 1.45a,b). Anteversion is likely to be present if internal rotation in extension exceeds 70 degrees and external rotation is less than 20 degrees. Graphs of the normal range with age are given in ▶ Fig. 1.45c,d.

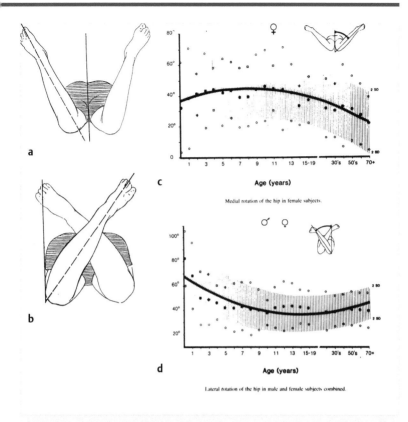

Fig. 1.45 Measurement technique and normal values for hip internal and external rotation in extension. (**a**) Measurement of internal rotation. (**b**) Measurement of external rotation. Hip rotation is usually measured in extension for assessment of torsion deformities. (**c**) Normal values for internal rotation with age. (**d**) Normal values for external rotation with age. (**c** and **d** are used with permission from Staheli LT, Corbett M, Wyss C, King H. Lower-extremity rotational problems in children. J Bone Joint Surg Am 1985;67(1):43 [Figs. 2C,D].)

1.5.10 Normal Radiographic Measurements of the Pediatric Foot

Radiographs are helpful in interpreting pathology in both the unoperated and the postoperative foot. The films should be taken with the patient standing, if possible. Normal values are given for the lateral talocalcaneal angle in ▶ Fig. 1.46 and the anteroposterior talocalcaneal angle in ▶ Fig. 1.47. Note that

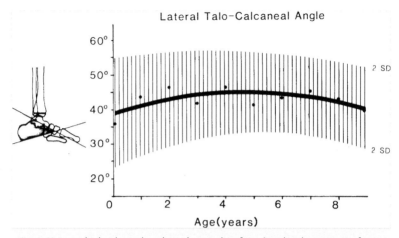

Fig. 1.46 Lateral talocalcaneal angle in the standing foot. (Used with permission from Vanderwilde R, Staheli LT, Chew DE, Malagon V. Measurements on radiographs of the foot in normal infants and children. J Bone Joint Surg Am 1988;70(3):410 [Fig. 2D].)

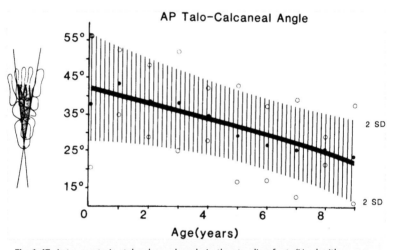

Fig. 1.47 Anteroposterior talocalcaneal angle in the standing foot. (Used with permission from Vanderwilde R, Staheli LT, Chew DE, Malagon V. Measurements on radiographs of the foot in normal infants and children. J Bone Joint Surg Am 1988;70 (3):409 [Fig. 2A].)

a decline in the value of both angles is seen with a varus foot (increasing parallelism), and an increase is seen with a valgus foot (increasing divergence).

1.6 Normal Gait in Children

Normal gait minimizes energy consumption. Gait deviations occur in response to a patient's neurologic or mechanical abnormalities. To understand gait by visual or laboratory analysis, it must be broken down into component characteristics.

1.6.1 Definitions

1. *Normal walking gait* is 60% *stance* and 40% *swing*; therefore, 20% is spent in *double support* (both limbs on the ground).
2. *Cadence*: Number of steps per unit of time.
3. *Stride*: One cycle, including right plus left steps.
4. *Kinematics*: Study of motion.
5. *Kinetics*: Study of forces that produce movement.
6. *Stance phase*: Period when one or both feet are on the ground.
7. *First rocker*: First stage of ankle motion in stance, from heel strike to foot flat; decelerates inertia of body; tibialis anterior contracts eccentrically.
8. *Second rocker*: Second stage of ankle motion in stance, from foot flat till heel rise; deceleration of tibia to relax quadriceps; soleus contracts eccentrically.
9. *Third rocker*: Third stage of ankle motion in stance, from heel rise till toe off; accelerates limb; gastrocnemius and soleus contract concentrically.
10. Phases of gait cycle (▶ Fig. 1.48; ▶ Fig. 1.49).

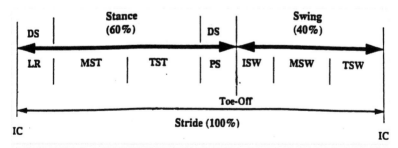

Fig. 1.48 Phases of gait cycle: DS, double support; IC, initial contact; LR, loading response; MS, midstance; TST, terminal stance; PS, preswing; ISW, initial swing; MSW, midswing; TSW, terminal swing.

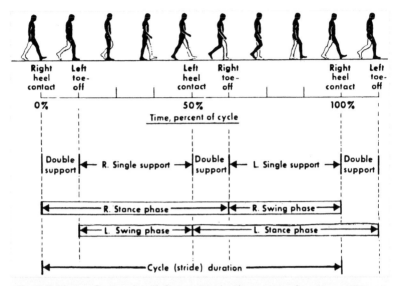

Fig. 1.49 Phases of gait cycle with figures. (Used with permission from Inman VT, Ralston HJ, Todd F. Human Walking. Baltimore, MD: Williams & Wilkins; 1981;26 [Fig. 2.6].)

1.6.2 Normal Parameters of Gait

1. Mature gait: Fully developed by age 7.
2. Velocity:
   a) 2-year-old: 0.78 m/s ± 0.2.
   b) 4-year-old: 1.0 m/s ± 0.2.
   c) 6-year-old: 1.1 m/s ± 0.2.
   d) Adult: 1.5 m/s ± 0.2.
3. Cadence:
   a) 2-year-old: 180 steps/min.
   b) 4-year-old: 160 steps/min.
   c) Adult: 116 steps/min.
4. Hip flexion: Extension 0 to 40 degrees during normal walking.
5. Knee flexion: Extension 5 to 60 degrees.
6. Ankle: 5 to 20 degrees plantarflexion (▶ Fig. 1.50 shows graphs of normal joint motion during gait).

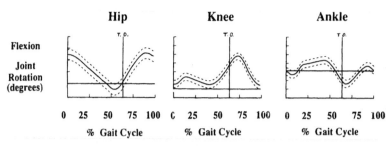

Fig. 1.50 Normal joint kinematics at the hip, knee, and ankle. (Used with permission from Gage JR. The clinical use of kinetics for evaluation of pathological gait in cerebral palsy. J Bone Joint Surg Am 1994;76(4):626 [Fig. 8, part I].)

1.6.3 Muscle Activity during Gait

1. Muscle activity may be measured by surface electrodes for large muscles or by fine wire electrodes for small muscles. A diagram of normal muscle activity is given in ► Fig. 1.51.
2. Muscle control by phase:
    a) Heel strike: Gluteus maximus, hamstrings, tibialis anterior.
    b) Loading response: Hamstrings, tibialis anterior, quadriceps, gluteus medius and maximus, adductor magnus.
    c) Midstance: Soleus, quadriceps, gluteus maximus.
    d) Terminal stance: Soleus, gastrocnemius, peroneal, toe flexors.
    e) Preswing: Gastrocnemius, adductor longus, rectus femoris.
    f) Initial swing: Hip flexors, tibialis anterior, toe extensors.
    g) Midswing: Tibialis anterior.
    h) Terminal swing: Hamstrings, quadriceps, tibialis anterior.

1.6.4 Evaluation of Patient with Gait Complaint/ Abnormality in Clinic

1. Full physical exam of lower limbs and trunk:
    a) Examine hip, knee, and ankle joints for full ROM. Examine for muscle spasticity, contracture, or extrapyramidal movements of lower limb.
    b) Neurologic exam of lower limb, including reflexes, motor strength, muscle tone, and sensory function.
    c) Radiographs to evaluate/document bone morphology, rotational deformities.
2. Systematically evaluate patient gait:
    a) Coronal plane: Instruct patient to walk away from you and back. Evaluate time spent on each limb and functional length of each limb. Note any

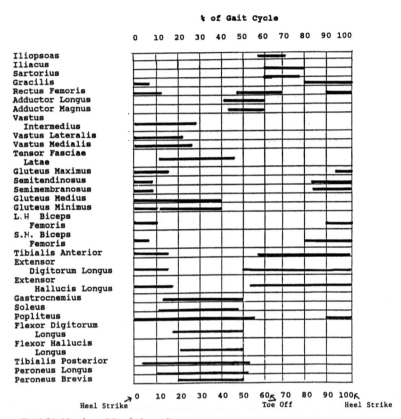

Fig. 1.51 Muscle activity during gait.

pelvic obliquity, trunk sway, hip adduction/abduction, or rotational abnormality. Observe each joint and portion of limb independently to isolate/document abnormality.

b) Sagittal plane: Instruct patient to walk perpendicular to your line of sight. Observe hip, knee, and ankle motion in sagittal plane, noting pelvic tilt, as well as hip/knee and ankle flexion/extension throughout gait cycle.

c) Document and quantify findings: Clearly document specific findings from clinical gait analysis. Quantification of findings is difficult in clinic: for more accurate and precise quantification, consider videotaped analysis or referral for gait analysis in motion laboratory.

1.6.5 Gait Analysis in Motion Laboratory

Gait analysis in motion laboratory captures patient motion by tracking 3D location of infrared markers placed on bony landmarks (excessive adiposity can decrease the utility/accuracy of gait analysis). Those locations are tracked over time and gait and can be used to reproduce patient kinematics. Muscle activation can be tracked by surface or fine wire EMGs. Force plate data also allow for kinetic analysis of patient movement. Gait analysis in a motion laboratory can assist in delineating the pathomechanics behind gait abnormalities that may have multiple causes.

Bibliography

1. Chambers HG, Sutherland DH. A practical guide to gait analysis. J Am Acad Orthop Surg 2002;10(3):222–231
2. Gage JR. The clinical use of kinetics for evaluation of pathological gait in cerebral palsy. J Bone Joint Surg Am 1994;76-A(4):622–631
3. Herzenberg JE, Standard S. Bone Ninja [an app for managing bone growth and angulation]. Available at: http://www.rubininstitute.com/RIAO/Bone-NinjaAppforiPad.aspx. Accessed June 20, 2018
4. Paley J, Talor J, Levin A, Bhave A, Paley D, Herzenberg JE. The multiplier method for prediction of adult height. J Pediatr Orthop 2004;24(6):732–737
5. Palmer F, Capute A. Keys to developmental assessment. In: McMillan J, ed. Oski's Pediatrics. 4th ed. Philadelphia, PA: Lippincott Williams & Wilkins; 2006:789

2 Disorders of Growth and Development in the Extremities

Paul D. Sponseller

2.1 Introduction

A summary of important pediatric conditions is provided in this and the following two chapters, focusing on concepts and key points. Principles and specific treatment details are covered more extensively in standard texts. Other major topics are covered in Chapter 5 (skeletal syndromes), Chapter 6 (neuromuscular disorders), and Chapter 7 (trauma) of this book.

2.2 Lower-Limb Length Inequality

2.2.1 Principles

1. Inequalities of lower-limb length of up to 1.0 to 1.5 cm are within normal variation of the population.
2. Inequalities of less than 2.5 cm do not cause back pain or noticeable limp.
3. Length inequalities are a much less common cause of limp than are joint disorders (contracture, pain) or muscle weakness.
4. The gait disturbance caused by inequality of limb length is usually subtle and consists of pelvic drop and compensatory knee flexion of the long limb and ankle equinus of the short limb.
5. Most congenital inequalities of limb length behave in a proportionate fashion with growth; that is, the ratio of the short leg to the long leg remains constant.

2.2.2 Congenital Causes

1. Congenital short femur, proximal focal femoral deficiency, tibial or fibular hemimelia, hemiatrophy, hemihypertrophy. Multiplier method predicts final discrepancy (see Chapter 1).
2. Systemic disorders: Ollier disease, fibrous dysplasia, osteochondromatosis, osteogenesis imperfecta, cerebral palsy. Multiplier method is not always predictive because of progressive deformity.

2.2.3 Acquired Causes

1. Developmental dysplasia of the hip (DDH; length difference resulting from growth disturbance or osteotomy).

2. Legg–Calvé–Perthes disease (may be up to 4 cm if proximal femoral physeal growth slows early).
3. Blount disease.
4. Trauma (fracture overlap, growth arrest).
5. Osteomyelitis with physeal arrest.
6. Foot deformities.

2.2.4 Measurement

1. Block method: Palpate height of iliac crests in standing patient. Add height to short limb by measured blocks until equal. This is a good screening method to determine whether further, more precise measurements are needed. Although not as precise for long bones as radiographic measurements, it does take into account all factors, such as contracture and shortening occurring within the foot or pelvis (▶ Fig. 2.1).

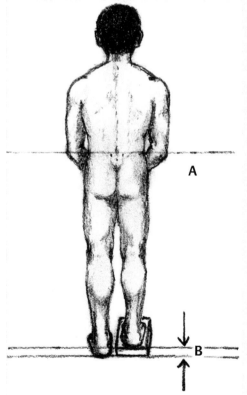

Fig. 2.1 The standing block test: a block is added under the short limb (B) until the pelvis is palpated to be level A.

2. Tape method: Measure from inferior margin of the anterior superior iliac spine (ASIS) to the medial malleolus. This method can be inaccurate in overweight patients or in those who have had anterior hip surgery and does not include foot discrepancies.
3. Scanogram: Images of hips, knees, and ankles are taken in one position alongside a radiographic ruler. This method does not account for foot discrepancies or contracture.
4. Computed radiograph: Computes lengths and angles of segments. This method may be used with low-dose radiography such as EOS.

2.2.5 Treatment

1. If discrepancy is less than 2.5 cm in a mature person, no treatment is needed.
2. 2.5 to ~4 cm: Leg lift or epiphyseodesis or shortening of corresponding long segment.
3. Approximately greater than 4 cm: Limb lengthening if no contraindications or combination of lengthening and shortening and lift.

Bibliography

1. Escott BG, Ravi B, Weathermon AC, et al. EOS low-dose radiography: a reliable and accurate upright assessment of lower-limb lengths. J Bone Joint Surg Am 2013;95(23):e1831–e1837
2. Paley D, Bhave A, Herzenberg JE, Bowen JR. Multiplier method for predicting limb-length discrepancy. J Bone Joint Surg Am 2000;82-A(10):1432–1446
3. Sabharwal S, Zhao C, McKeon JJ, McClemens E, Edgar M, Behrens F. Computed radiographic measurement of limb-length discrepancy. Full-length standing anteroposterior radiograph compared with scanogram. J Bone Joint Surg Am 2006;88(10):2243–2251

2.3 Developmental Dysplasia of the Hip

2.3.1 Principles

Developmental dysplasia of the hip is caused by forces acting on the hip in utero. The risk is increased by abnormalities of connective tissue. DDH is a spectrum, from hips that are subluxatable or dislocatable (Barlow positive) to dislocated (Ortolani positive). The combined incidence is 2 to 5 per 1,000.

All hips should be physically screened by a knowledgeable examiner at birth and again within the first few months of life. The infant should be made as quiet and comfortable as possible for the examination, using warmth, contact, low light, feeding, or a pacifier. Abnormal physical signs that are marked with an asterisk (*) below should prompt reexamination or ultrasound, with treatment if these are abnormal.

2.3.2 Risk Factors in History

The following factors increase the risk of hip dysplasia in descending order and should prompt reexamination or ultrasound:
1. Positive family history of DDH.
2. Breech position at the end of gestation (5% are unstable). A breech female should have a screening ultrasound.

2.3.3 Physical Examination for Developmental Hip Dysplasia in the Newborn

1. Appearance at rest: The dysplastic hip is more adducted at rest in unilateral cases and may have a deeper or extra high fold proximally.
2. *Asymmetric passive abduction: Dislocated hip will lack passive abduction compared with the normal side (▸ Fig. 2.2a).
3. *The Barlow test will cause pistoning of the proximal femur if dislocatable (▸ Fig. 2.2b).
4. *The Ortolani test will cause a "clunk" as a dislocated hip is relocated. Examine each hip separately; stabilize the pelvis with the other hand (▸ Fig. 2.2c). The Ortolani and Barlow tests are for *translation* of the femur. A "click" per se is not a positive test; only 1% of patients with a click have dysplasia. A click may come from the patella or the meniscus of the knee as well as from the fascia lata or a synovial fold in the hip.
5. Proximal location of greater trochanters is a helpful sign in diagnosing a patient with bilateral irreducible hip dislocations. Also, the femoral head may cause a prominence superiorly.
6. Significant foot deformity or torticollis may increase the risk of hip dysplasia and should prompt a careful examination of the hips.

2.3.4 Evaluation of the Older Child for Developmental Dysplasia of the Hip

In the older child with hip dysplasia, the signs progressively change. Reducibility of the hip in the awake patient is lost after about 3 months, and one must rely more on indirect signs:
1. Asymmetric passive abduction.

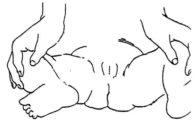

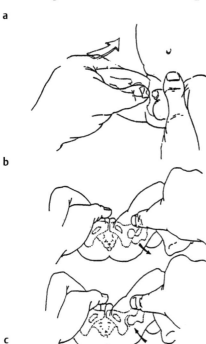

Fig. 2.2 (**a**) Asymmetric abduction; left side is dysplastic. (**b**) Barlow test (done on one hip at a time). (**c**) Ortolani test.

a

b

c

2. Galeazzi test will show thigh shortening on the side that is dislocated (▶ Fig. 2.3a). The pelvis should be kept horizontal during this test.
3. Leg-length discrepancy.
4. Trendelenburg gait.
5. Palpable femoral head posterior to the acetabulum.
6. Nélaton line (an imaginary line between the ASIS and the ischium) should project superior to the trochanter (▶ Fig. 2.3b).
7. Klisic line between the greater trochanter and the ASIS should project cephalad to the umbilicus (▶ Fig. 2.3c).

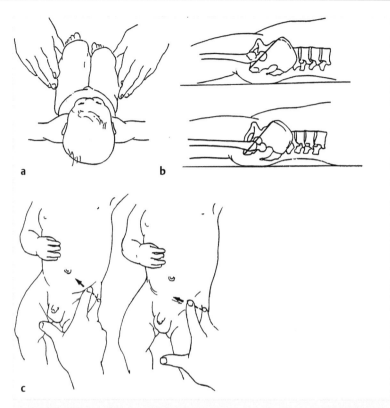

Fig. 2.3 (a) Galeazzi sign shows apparent thigh shortening on dysplastic side (right). (b) If dislocated, the greater trochanter will lie proximal to Nélaton line (anterior superior iliac spine to ischium). (c) Klisic line in the normal hip falls above the umbilicus.

8. Increased lumbar lordosis in stance (if bilateral) is due to posterior displacement and mechanical disadvantage of hip abductors.

2.3.5 Imaging

Ultrasonography

The role of ultrasound in the diagnosis of dysplasia varies regionally. Its benefit is its ability to show cartilage and other soft tissues, as well as observe stability in response to stress. Interpretation of an ultrasound considers both static and dynamic findings.

The ultrasound view is named according to the *direction of the transducer*: transverse or coronal—and the *position of the hip*: neutral or flexion. The highest frequency possible (3–7 MHz) will give the best resolution, but this must usually be reduced with age to obtain adequate penetration.

Coronal View

In this view, the landmarks are similar to those seen on a plain radiograph, when the transducer is in the mid acetabular plane. By convention, the lateral wall of the ilium is displayed horizontally.

1. The stability and gross appearance are the most important features.
2. The following other parameters should be checked (▶ Fig. 2.4):
   a) Femoral head coverage: The percent of the femoral head medial to the outer line of the ilium. This should be greater than 50%.
   b) Alpha angle, or acetabular roof line, between the lateral ilium and the bony acetabular roof. It is analogous to the acetabular index and should be greater than 60 degrees.
   c) Beta angle, or slope of the labrum versus the lateral wall of the ilium. It should be less than 55 degrees, indicating a downward slope of the labrum.

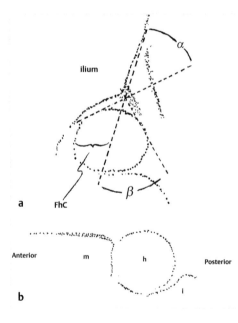

Fig. 2.4 Drawings of ultrasound images. (**a**) Coronal view. FhC, femoral head coverage; α angle, acetabular roof line; β angle, slope of labrum. (**b**) Transverse view. Note the "U" formed by the metaphysis and the acetabulum. h, head of femur; i, ischium; m, metaphysis of femur.

Transverse View

In this view, the hip is flexed and the transducer is placed posterolaterally in the transverse plane of the body. The combination of echoes from the femoral metaphysis and the acetabulum normally form a "U." When dislocated, the femoral head comes to lie lateral and posterior to the acetabulum, and the U is disrupted.

Radiographic Evaluation

1. Grades of hip dislocation according to Tönnis indicate the position of the ossific nucleus relative to the Perkin vertical line (p) and the Hilgenreiner horizontal line (h) (▶ Fig. 2.5):
   a) Nucleus medial to Perkin line.
   b) Nucleus lateral to Perkin line.
   c) Nucleus at Hilgenreiner line.
   d) Nucleus above Hilgenreiner line.
2. The *acetabular index* is the angle formed between the Hilgenreiner line and the inner and outer borders of the acetabular roof (▶ Fig. 2.6a, right hip). It is useful in assessing hip development in early years, before the center of the femoral head can be accurately identified. The normal values are shown in ▶ Fig. 2.6b.
3. Center edge angle (CEA) of Wiberg:
   a) CEA measures the coverage of the femoral head by the acetabulum (▶ Fig. 2.6a, left hip). Long-term follow-up studies by Wiberg have shown a correlation between development of symptoms after maturity and CEA below 20 degrees.

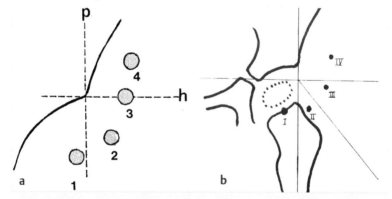

Fig. 2.5 (a) Tonnis grades of hip dislocation based upon position of femoral epiphysis. p, perkins line; h, horizontal line at outer edge of acetabulum. **(b)** For young patients who do not have an ossific nucleus, the IHDI (international hip dysplasia institute) grades are used, referencing the femoral metaphysis.

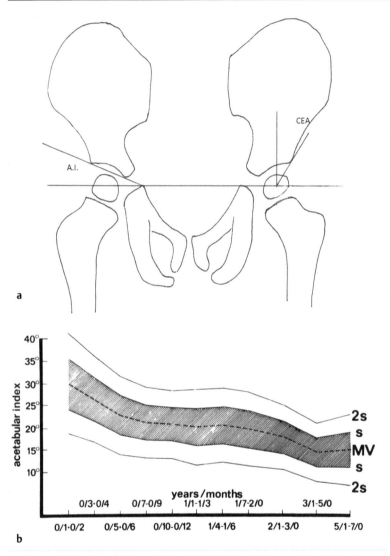

Fig. 2.6 (a) Acetabular index (A.I.) measurement (right hip) and measurement of center edge angle (CEA) of Wiberg (left hip). **(b)** Acetabular index normal values for age. MV, mean value; s, one standard deviation; 2s, two standard deviations. **(b** is used with permission from Tonnis D. Normal values of the hip joint for the evaluation of x-rays in children and adults. Clin Orthop Relat Res 1976;119:41 (Fig. 2).)

b) Normal values—lower limit of normal:
1. 5 to 8 years: 19 degrees.
2. 9 to 12 years: 25 degrees.
3. 13: 26 degrees.
4. Less precise under 5 years.

Bibliography

1. Tönnis D. Normal values of the hip joint for the evaluation of X-rays in children and adults. Clin Orthop Relat Res 1976;(119):39–47

2.3.6 Management of Hip Dysplasia

▶ Fig. 2.7 is a general algorithm for the management of dysplasia. Guidelines given may be modified based on individual factors.

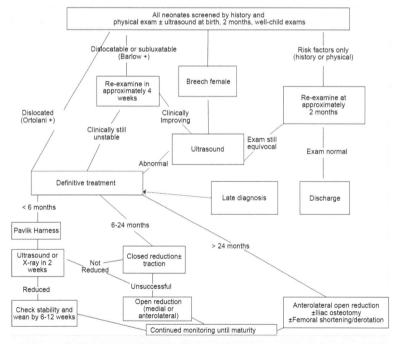

Fig. 2.7 General algorithm for the management of pediatric hip dysplasia.

Bibliography

1. Grissom L, Harcke HT, Thacker M. Imaging in the surgical management of developmental dislocation of the hip. Clin Orthop Relat Res 2008;466(4):791–801

2. Guille JT, Pizzutillo PD, MacEwen GD. Development dysplasia of the hip from birth to six months. J Am Acad Orthop Surg 2000;8(4):232–242

3. Sankar WN, Nduaguba A, Flynn JM. Ilfeld abduction orthosis is an effective second-line treatment after failure of Pavlik harness for infants with developmental dysplasia of the hip. J Bone Joint Surg Am 2015;97(4):292–297

4. Shin CH, Yoo WJ, Park MS, Kim JH, Choi IH, Cho TJ. Acetabular remodeling and role of osteotomy after closed reduction of developmental dysplasia of the hip. J Bone Joint Surg Am 2016;98(11):952–957

5. Tennant SJ, Eastwood DM, Calder P, Hashemi-Nejad A, Catterall A. A protocol for the use of closed reduction in children with developmental dysplasia of the hip incorporating open psoas and adductor releases and a short-leg cast: mid-term outcomes in 113 hips. Bone Joint J 2016;98-B(11):1548–1553

2.4 Legg–Calvé–Perthes Disease

Legg–Calvé–Perthes disease (idiopathic avascular necrosis [AVN] of the immature femoral head) is most commonly seen in children aged 4 to 10 years. Five percent of patients develop bilateral involvement, but this is usually at different times (asynchronous). Synchronous involvement should suggest the possibility of skeletal dysplasia, hypothyroidism, or steroid use.

2.4.1 Symptoms

1. Minimal or no history of trauma.
2. Stiffness.
3. Intermittent mild pain or no pain at all.

2.4.2 Signs

1. Mild Trendelenburg gait.
2. No pain with gentle motion.
3. Limitation of abduction and internal rotation.

2.4.3 Imaging

1. Chronological sequence (Waldenstrom; ▶ Fig. 2.8):
   I) Sclerosis of epiphysis:
   a) No loss of height.
   b) Loss of height.

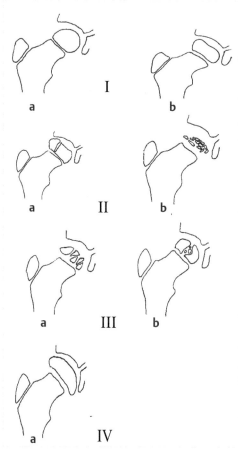

Fig. 2.8 Waldenstrom chronologic stages of Perthes: I, sclerosis of epiphysis; II, fragmentation; III, early healing; IV, complete healing.

II) Fragmentation:
  a) One to two fissures.
  b) Advanced fragmentation.
III) Early healing:
  a) Early new bone laterally.
  b) New bone greater than one-third of epiphysis.
IV) Complete healing.
2. Staging:
  a) Catterall (▶ Fig. 2.9):
    1. Central anterior involvement of head only.

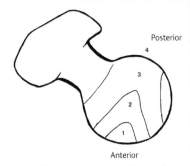

Fig. 2.9 Catterall classification of Perthes disease as viewed from above.

Posterior

4

3

2

1

Anterior

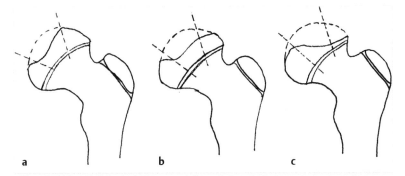

a   b   c

Fig. 2.10 (a–c) Herring lateral pillar classification of Perthes.

2. Greater central head involvement but intact medial and lateral column.
3. Lateral three quarters of femoral head involved with only intact medial column; metaphyseal reaction.
4. Whole-head involvement, with metaphyseal reaction and remodeling of epiphysis.

b) Herring lateral pillar classification predicts flattening during healing (▶ Fig. 2.10):

1. Lateral pillar is intact without radiographic change.
2. Lateral pillar is collapsed, but height is still greater than 50%.
3. Lateral pillar is collapsed to less than 50% of original height.

3. Prognostic signs:

a) "Head-at-risk signs" of Catterall:

1. Lateral calcification.
2. Lateral subluxation.

3. Gage sign: lucency proximal and distal to lateral physis.
4. Metaphyseal reaction.
5. Horizontal physis (meaning limb is adducted).

b) Epiphyseal extrusion (▶ Fig. 2.11) greater than 20% carries poor long-term prognosis.

c) Mose sphericity: Deviation of head periphery from a perfect sphere by more than 3 mm on anteroposterior (AP) and lateral radiograph carries poor long-term prognosis.

d) Stulberg rating (used after healing) assesses femoral head sphericity and its congruency with the acetabulum. There are five different stages; these have been correlated with long-term outcome (▶ Fig. 2.12).

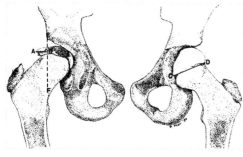

Fig. 2.11 Measurement of epiphyseal extrusion = a-b / c-d. (Used with permission from Green NE, Beauchamp RD, Griffin PP. Epiphyseal extrusion as a prognostic index in Legg-Calve-Perthes disease. J Bone Joint Surg Am 1981;63 (6):902 (Fig. 1).)

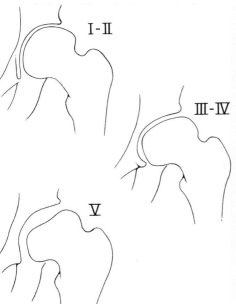

Fig. 2.12 Stulberg rating of outcome of healed Perthes. Stages I and II are spherical and congruent and have a low likelihood of degenerative joint disease. Stages III and IV are aspherical and congruous and have a risk of degenerative joint disease by middle age. Stage V is aspherical and incongruous, and there is a risk of degenerative joint disease before age 50 years. (Used with permission from Stulberg SD, Cooperman DR, Wallensten R. The natural history of Legg-Calve-Perthes disease. J Bone Joint Surg Am 1981;63(7):1095–1108.)

4. Arthrogram, magnetic resonance imaging (MRI): These are not routinely indicated but may be helpful in selected cases. Perfusion MRI may help establish degree of AVN.

2.4.4 Differential Diagnosis

1. Hypothyroidism.
2. Multiple epiphyseal dysplasias.
3. Spondyloepiphyseal dysplasia.
4. Meyer dysplasia (bilateral synchronous early childhood AVN; better prognosis).
5. Storage disorder (Gaucher disease, mucopolysaccharidoses).
6. AVN following trauma, steroids, sickle cell infarct, DDH treatment.

2.4.5 Treatment

1. There is no consensus on a protocol. However, many hips have a poor long-term outcome, and some hips appear to be helped by treatment. Containment is indicated if several of the following features are present:
   a) Head involvement greater than 50% (Catterall 3–4, Herring B or B/C border).
   b) Age over 8 years.
   c) No collapse or extrusion.
2. Containment options:
   a) Abduction brace or Petrie casts.
   b) Femoral varus osteotomy.
   c) Iliac rotational osteotomy or augmentation.
   d) Combinations of b and c.
3. Late options:
   a) Epiphysiodesis for leg length inequality greater than 2 cm.
   b) Valgus osteotomy for symptomatic hinge abduction.
   c) Trochanteric transfer for persistent abductor weakness.
   d) Epiphyseal osteotomy for femoral incongruity.

Bibliography

1. Herring JA, Kim HT, Browne R. Legg-Calve-Perthes disease. Part I: Classification of radiographs with use of the modified lateral pillar and Stulberg classifications. J Bone Joint Surg Am 2004;86-A(10):2103–2120
2. Herring JA, Kim HT, Browne R. Legg-Calve-Perthes disease. Part II: Prospective multicenter study of the effect of treatment on outcome. J Bone Joint Surg Am 2004;86-A(10):2121–2134

3. Hyman JE, Trupia EP, Wright ML, et al; International Perthes Study Group Members. Interobserver and intraobserver reliability of the modified Waldenström classification system for staging of Legg-Calvé-Perthes disease. J Bone Joint Surg Am 2015;97(8):643–650
4. Joseph B, Nair NS, Narasimha Rao K, Mulpuri K, Varghese G. Optimal timing for containment surgery for Perthes disease. J Pediatr Orthop 2003;23 (5):601–606

2.5 Transient Synovitis of the Hip

2.5.1 Overview

1. Transient synovitis of the hip is characterized by the acute onset of monarticular hip pain, limp, and restricted motion.
2. It is the most common cause of hip pain in children.
3. Child is usually 1 to 4 years of age, but any age can be affected.
4. Synovitis must be distinguished from septic arthritis (Kocher's clinical practice guideline).
5. Gradual but complete resolution over several days to weeks is the norm.
6. Cause is unknown, but it may be immune mediated.

2.5.2 Diagnosis

1. A diagnosis of exclusion.
2. Acute onset of unilateral hip pain in an otherwise healthy child; often after respiratory illness.
3. The patient may be afebrile or have a low-grade fever.
4. Laboratory values are nonspecific and are often within normal limits.
5. Kocher's criteria to distinguish septic arthritis from transient synovitis:
   a) Refusal to bear weight.
   b) Temperature greater than 38.
   c) WBC greater than 12,000.
   d) ESR greater than 40.

2.5.3 Physical Examination

1. Limp and antalgic gait are common.
2. Most patients can bear weight on the involved extremity with assistance.
3. Hip is held in a flexed, externally rotated position. Restricted range of motion, especially abduction and rotation; slow movement is better.
4. Pain is not as great as with septic arthritis.

2.5.4 Laboratory Tests

1. Laboratory tests are usually nonspecific and within normal limits, but they may help rule out other diagnoses.
2. Peripheral WBC count is normal to slightly elevated.
3. ESR averages 20 mm/hour but may be slightly higher.
4. Blood culture, rheumatoid factor, and Lyme titers results are usually within normal limits.
5. Aspiration of joint fluid is not needed if presentation is typical. If done, results are nonspecific.

2.5.5 Imaging

1. Plain films of the hip: AP and lateral views.
2. In transient synovitis, they are normal but can help rule out other diagnoses.
3. Ultrasound may be used to assess for effusion and to guide aspiration if infection cannot be ruled out clinically.
4. MRI is needed only in cases of persistent pain.

2.5.6 Differential Diagnosis

1. Septic arthritis.
2. Osteomyelitis in the femoral neck or pelvis.
3. Tuberculous arthritis.
4. Psoas abscess.
5. Other muscle infection about the hip.
6. Juvenile rheumatoid arthritis.
7. Idiopathic chondrolysis.
8. Acute rheumatic fever.
9. Legg–Calvé–Perthes disease.
10. Tumor.
11. Sacroiliac joint infection.

2.5.7 Treatment

1. Bed rest at home if diagnosis is clear, or in hospital if further workup is needed.
2. Nonsteroidal anti-inflammatory drugs (NSAIDs).
3. Prompt improvement should be seen: if not, then look for other diagnoses.
4. Activity as tolerated when clinically improved.

2.5.8 Prognosis

Good; no clear evidence of increased risk of AVN.

Bibliography

1. Dobbs Matthew B. Transient synovitis of the hip. In: Morrissy RT, Weinstein SL, eds. Lovell and Winter's Pediatric Orthopaedics. Vol. 2. 6th ed. Philadelphia, PA: Lippincott Williams & Wilkins; 2006:1142–1147
2. Haueisen DC, Weiner DS, Weiner SD. The characterization of "transient synovitis of the hip" in children. J Pediatr Orthop 1986;6(1):11–17
3. Johnson K, Haigh SF, Ehtisham S, Ryder C, Gardner-Medwin J. Childhood idiopathic chondrolysis of the hip: MRI features. Pediatr Radiol 2003;33 (3):194–199
4. Kocher MS, Mandiga R, Murphy JM, et al. A clinical practice guideline for treatment of septic arthritis in children: efficacy in improving process of care and effect on outcome of septic arthritis of the hip. J Bone Joint Surg Am 2003;85-A(6):994–999
5. Kocher MS, Mandiga R, Zurakowski D, Barnewolt C, Kasser JR. Validation of a clinical prediction rule for the differentiation between septic arthritis and transient synovitis of the hip in children. J Bone Joint Surg Am 2004;86-A (8):1629–1635
6. Landin LA, Danielsson LG, Wattsgård C. Transient synovitis of the hip. Its incidence, epidemiology and relation to Perthes' disease. J Bone Joint Surg Br 1987;69(2):238–242

2.6 Slipped Capital Femoral Epiphysis

2.6.1 Background

1. Incidence: 2 to 10 per 100,000:
   a) Higher rate in males than in females.
   b) Higher in African Americans.
   c) 20% of patients have bilateral involvement at presentation.
   d) 20% of patients become more bilateral later.
2. Etiologic factors:
   a) Obesity.
   b) Trauma: Mild or severe.
   c) Endocrine disorders: Hypothyroidism, hypogonadism, rickets, renal failure.
   d) Down syndrome.
   e) Family history.
   f) Radiation.

2.6.2 Classification

1. Loder classification:
   a) Stable: Able to bear weight (even with crutches).
   b) Unstable: Unable to bear weight.
2. Chronological:
   a) Acute: Symptoms of less than 3 weeks' duration.
   b) Chronic: Symptoms for 3 weeks or longer.
3. Severity:
   a) Grade I: Less than 33% slip of epiphysis on metaphysis.
   b) Grade II: 33 to 50% slip.
   c) Grade III: More than 50% slip.
   d) "Pre-slip": Symptoms are present in patient at risk, but no observable slip is seen; MRI may be positive.

2.6.3 Clinical Presentation

1. Age 9 to 14 years, most common.
2. Antalgic limp.
3. Pain in the thigh, knee, or hip.
4. Leg externally rotated during gait and at rest.
5. Internal rotation less in flexion than in extension.
6. Seasonal variation: Highest rates in September, lowest in March because of sunlight and vitamin D cycles (delayed effects).
7. Age–weight test: If younger than 10 or older than 16 years or weight is less than 50th percentile, then suspect nonidiopathic slip and perform an endocrine workup.
8. Height test: If height is below 10th percentile for age, risk of atypical slip is increased, perform an endocrine workup.

2.6.4 Imaging

1. Slip is best seen on lateral view.
2. AP view:
   a) Physeal widening, irregularity.
   b) Decreased epiphyseal height.
   c) "Klein line": Line on lateral femoral neck with slipped capital femoral epiphysis (SCFE) transects less than 20% of epiphysis in child older than 10 years.
   d) Chondrolysis-joint space narrowing may be seen before treatment (rare).

2.6.5 Treatment

1. Immediate weight relief (bed rest).
2. Traction for acute slip for comfort or reduction if severe (optional).
3. Fixation in situ:
   a) Single screw is centrally placed within physis.
   b) Second screw may be used if first is not perfect or if slip is severe.
4. Realignment: Main indication is the patient who is dissatisfied with limb deformity resulting from slip; it is not commonly needed.
   a) Open realignment and pinning of acute slip (± surgical dislocation).
   b) Cuneiform osteotomy just below physis.
   c) Base of neck osteotomy: some series show high AVN rate.
   d) Subtrochanteric osteotomy (Southwick).
5. Prophylactic contralateral pinning:
   a) Cost–benefit studies show prophylactic pinning is justifiable (at the surgeon's discretion).
   b) Main indication is a patient in whom diagnosis of late contralateral SCFE may be missed as a result of impaired communication or follow-up.
   c) Also valid option in patients with SCFE before growth spurt (in girls younger than 10 years, in boys younger than 12 years).
   d) If triradiate cartilage is closed or in a girl older than 13 years or in a boy older than 14 years, then there is a low risk of subsequent slip (~7%).

2.6.6 Complications

1. Chondrolysis: Affects 5% or less and usually improves with time and physical therapy.
2. AVN:
   a) Greater in unstable or acute slips.
   b) May be focal or complete.
   c) Some healing is possible in young patients.
   d) Some patients can function for 10 to 20 years with AVN before salvage is needed.

Bibliography

1. Carney BT, Weinstein SL, Noble J. Long-term follow-up of slipped capital femoral epiphysis. J Bone Joint Surg Am 1991;73(5):667–674
2. Escott BG, De La Rocha A, Jo CH, Sucato DJ, Karol LA. Patient-reported health outcomes after in situ percutaneous fixation for slipped capital femoral epiphysis: an average twenty-year follow-up study. J Bone Joint Surg Am 2015;97(23):1929–1934

3. Kocher MS, Bishop JA, Hresko MT, Millis MB, Kim YJ, Kasser JR. Prophylactic pinning of the contralateral hip after unilateral slipped capital femoral epiphysis. J Bone Joint Surg Am 2004;86-A(12):2658–2665

4. Koenig KM, Thomson JD, Anderson KL, Carney BT. Does skeletal maturity predict sequential contralateral involvement after fixation of slipped capital femoral epiphysis? J Pediatr Orthop 2007;27(7):796–800

5. Loder RT, Aronsson DD, Weinstein SL, Breur GJ, Ganz R, Leunig M. Slipped capital femoral epiphysis. Instr Course Lect 2008;57:473–498

6. Loder RT, Starnes T, Dikos G. Atypical and typical (idiopathic) slipped capital femoral epiphysis. Reconfirmation of the age-weight test and description of the height and age-height tests. J Bone Joint Surg Am 2006;88(7):1574–1581

7. Riad J, Bajelidze G, Gabos PG. Bilateral slipped capital femoral epiphysis: predictive factors for contralateral slip. J Pediatr Orthop 2007;27(4):411–414

8. Schrader T, Jones CR, Kaufman AM, Herzog MM. Intraoperative monitoring of epiphyseal perfusion in slipped capital femoral epiphysis. J Bone Joint Surg Am 2016;98(12):1030–1040

9. Schultz WR, Weinstein JN, Weinstein SL, Smith BG. Prophylactic pinning of the contralateral hip in slipped capital femoral epiphysis: evaluation of long-term outcome for the contralateral hip with use of decision analysis. J Bone Joint Surg Am 2002;84-A(8):1305–1314

10. Yildirim Y, Bautista S, Davidson RS. Chondrolysis, osteonecrosis, and slip severity in patients with subsequent contralateral slipped capital femoral epiphysis. J Bone Joint Surg Am 2008;90(3):485–492

2.7 Developmental Coxa Vara

A varus deformity of the femoral neck that is usually progressive. Incidence is 1 in 25,000. Thirty percent of cases are bilateral.

2.7.1 Imaging

1. Femoral neck shortened and in varus.
2. Inverted **Y** appearance of physis represents a shear plane through metaphysis.
3. Triangular fragment on inferior femoral neck.
4. Decreased femoral anteversion.
5. Mild acetabular dysplasia.

2.7.2 Signs and Symptoms

1. Abnormal gait caused by abductor weakness and leg-length inequality.

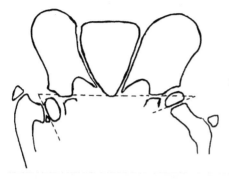

Hilgenreiner's-epiphyseal Angle

Normal= Less than 25°

Fig. 2.13 Hilgenreiner–epiphyseal angle; normal is less than 25 degrees. Note "inverted Y" appearance of physis on involved right hip.

2. Activity-related hip pain.
3. Length inequality if unilateral: usually less than 2.5 cm.

2.7.3 Differential Diagnosis

1. Cleidocranial dysplasia.
2. Metaphyseal dysplasia.
3. Morquio syndrome.
4. Idiopathic.

2.7.4 Treatment

1. Observe if Hilgenreiner–epiphyseal angle is less than 45 degrees (▶ Fig. 2.13).
2. Valgus-derotation osteotomy if greater than 45 degrees and progressive and symptomatic if greater than 60 degrees at diagnosis.

Bibliography

1. Weinstein JN, Kuo KN, Millar EA. Congenital coxa vara. A retrospective review. J Pediatr Orthop 1984;4(1):70–77

2.8 Proximal Focal Femoral Deficiency

A spectrum of congenital femoral anomalies including a temporary or permanent discontinuity in the proximal femur.

2.8.1 Classification (Aitken; See ▶ Fig. 2.14)

1. A: Femur is in continuity but appears discontinuous early.
2. B: Varus/shortening is more extreme, but most ossify later.
3. C: Small acetabulum but no femoral head.
4. D: No femoral head or acetabulum.

Other classification systems exist but are less widely used.

2.8.2 Characteristics

1. 15% are bilateral (most type D).
2. More than 50% have other lower extremity anomalies, most commonly fibular hemimelia.
3. Affected limb is a constant proportion to the length of the normal limb.

2.8.3 Problems

1. Limb-length inequality (if unilateral).
2. Pelvic-femoral instability.
3. Malrotation of lower extremity (flexion–abduction–external rotation).
4. Proximal muscle weakness.

2.8.4 Treatment

1. Bilateral:
   a) Patients walk without prostheses if feet are all right.
   b) Nonfunctional feet may need surgery.
   c) Extension prostheses may be used when desired to increase height.
2. Unilateral:
   a) Hip abnormalities: Valgus osteotomy and lengthening for types A and B; consider femoropelvic arthrodesis for type D versus containment of thigh segment in a prosthesis.
   b) Knee: Offer rotationplasty if foot and ankle are strong and positioned distal to the contralateral knee. Syme disarticulation is another option. Both are combined with fusion of anatomic knee to increase lever arm.
   c) Foot: Prosthesis equalizes length and provides plantigrade foot (▶ Fig. 2.14).

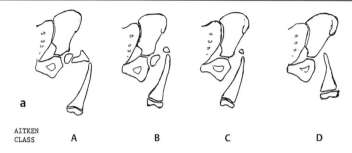

AITKEN
CLASS   A   B   C   D

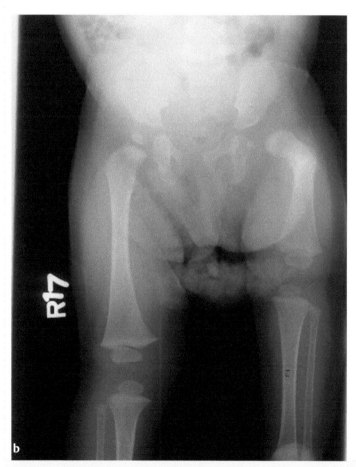

Fig. 2.14 (a) Proximal focal femoral deficiency: Aitken classification. (b) Radiographic image of Aitken Class A.

Bibliography

1. Aitken GT. Proximal Femoral Focal Deficiency: Definition, Classification and Management. National Academy of Sciences Symposium, Washington, DC; 1969
2. Fowler EG, Hester DM, Oppenheim WL, Setoguchi Y, Zernicke RF. Contrasts in gait mechanics of individuals with proximal femoral focal deficiency: Syme amputation versus Van Nes rotational osteotomy. J Pediatr Orthop 1999;19(6):720–731
3. Kalamchi A, Cowell HR, Kim KI. Congenital deficiency of the femur. J Pediatr Orthop 1985;5(2):129–134
4. Pappas AM. Congenital abnormalities of the femur and related lower extremity malformations: classification and treatment. J Pediatr Orthop 1983;3(1):45–60

2.9 Bladder Exstrophy

A spectrum of anomalies that may involve the bladder, pelvis, intestinal tract, and external genitalia.
1. The *most common* form is "classic" exstrophy, which involves a widened pelvis with an anterior diastasis, an open bladder, and a complete epispadias.
2. The *mildest* form is epispadias, which may have a closed bladder but widened pelvic symphysis.
3. The *most pronounced* expression of this spectrum is cloacal exstrophy, which usually involves all of the above as well as omphalocele and a lumbosacral neural tube defect. It often includes anomalies of the spine and extremities.
4. The incidence of bladder exstrophy is around 1:25,000 live births. Males are more commonly affected.

2.9.1 Clinical Features

1. Defect in the lower abdominal wall.
2. Open bladder and urethra.
3. In cloacal exstrophy, the abdominal wall defect is larger and the lower intestinal tract is exposed.
4. A spinal and a neurologic examination should be performed. Often in cloacal patients, there is lipomeningocele or myelomeningocele. Hip dislocation, foot deformity, or partial sacral agenesis may occur.

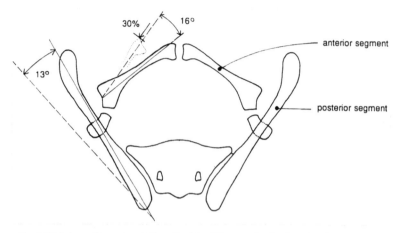

Fig. 2.15 Schematic representation of pelvic differences in classic exstrophy versus normal in the transverse plane.

2.9.2 Imaging

There is separation of pubic bones, typically about 4 to 5 cm at birth, and it increases steadily with age (▶ Fig. 2.15). The iliac wings are externally rotated and "flattened." The ischiopubic bones are slightly underdeveloped. The hips themselves rarely show dysplasia.

2.9.3 Treatment

1. The urologist usually performs the reconstruction in stages, including closure of the bladder and lower abdominal wall soon after birth, followed by epispadias closure at the same time or at a later date. Surgery to achieve continence is commonly performed after the age at which children are normally continent and may consist of bladder neck suspension.
2. Orthopaedic surgery of the pelvic deformity is indicated only if it is needed to achieve urologic goals.
3. In the neonatal period, the pubis may be approximated manually and temporarily held with suturing.
4. In an older child, iliac osteotomy is indicated either anteriorly or posteriorly.

2.9.4 Prognosis

The hip function in the untreated patient with classic bladder exstrophy is good. Children walk at a normal age, although they have an increased external foot-progression angle. This becomes less pronounced over time. Adults with exstrophy have an increased incidence of pain in the region of the sacroiliac joints. One natural history study suggests an increased incidence of degenerative disease of the hip in patients with uncorrected exstrophy. Patients with exstrophy are usually fertile.

Bibliography

1. Aadalen RJ, O'Phelan EH, Chisholm TC, McParland FA Jr, Sweetser TH Jr. Exstrophy of the bladder: long-term results of bilateral posterior iliac osteotomies and two-stage anatomic repair. Clin Orthop Relat Res 1980;151 (151):193–200
2. Jani MM, Sponseller PD, Gearhart JP, Barrance PJ, Genda E, Chao EY. The hip in adults with classic bladder exstrophy: a biomechanical analysis. J Pediatr Orthop 2000;20(3):296–301
3. Okubadejo GO, Sponseller PD, Gearhart JP. Complications in orthopedic management of exstrophy. J Pediatr Orthop 2003;23(4):522–528
4. Sponseller PD, Bisson LJ, Gearhart JP, Jeffs RD, Magid D, Fishman E. The anatomy of the pelvis in the exstrophy complex. J Bone Joint Surg Am 1995;77 (2):177–189
5. Sponseller PD, Jani MM, Jeffs RD, Gearhart JP. Anterior innominate osteotomy in repair of bladder exstrophy. J Bone Joint Surg Am 2001;83-A(2):184–193

2.10 Tibia Vara

A focal varus deformity of the proximal tibia resulting from overload causing disordered medial growth. Tibia vara may have onset in the infantile, juvenile, or adolescent period (▶ Table 2.1).

2.10.1 Imaging

1. Normal alignment of the lower extremity is shown in Chapter 1 (Fig. 1.40).
2. In infantile tibia vara, changes involve physeal depression with lucency and beaking of the corresponding metaphysis and epiphysis. These changes have been staged 1 through 7 by Langenskjold (▶ Fig. 2.16).
3. Infants younger than 2 years have inadequate ossification to assign Langenskjold stages. As an alternate means of early diagnosis, the metaphyseal–diaphyseal angle (MDA) is drawn (▶ Fig. 2.17). MDA greater than 16 degrees is diagnostic of infantile Blount disease; MDA less than 11 degrees is normal; and MDA between 11 and 15 degrees is indeterminate and should be monitored.

Table 2.1 Comparison of types of tibia vara (by age)

Parameter	Infantile (0–3 y)	Juvenile (3–10 y)	Adolescent (11 y and older)
Pain	No	No	Usually
Site of varus	Proximal tibia only; medial tibia plateau may be tilted or depressed. Femur often in valgus	Tibia	Distal femur and proximal tibia in varus
Risk of bar	Yes	No	No
Treatment	Observe or brace; hemiepiphysiodesis if mild; osteotomy of femur and tibia as indicated; may need lengthening later	hemiepiphyseodesis or osteotomy	Hemiepiphysiodesis if mild, growing Osteotomy of femur and tibia

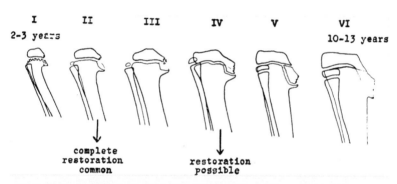

Fig. 2.16 Langenskjold stages of infantile tibia vara. (Used with permission from Langenskjold A. Tibia vara (osteochondrosis deformans tibiae): a survey of 23 cases. Acta Chir Scand 1952;103(1):1–22 (Fig. 5).)

4. Medial physeal slope greater than 60 degrees may predict recurrent bowing after osteotomy (▶ Fig. 2.18).
5. Medial plateau depression greater than 30 degrees may be seen in neglected infantile tibia vara (▶ Fig. 2.19).
6. Mechanical axis deviation quantifies the degree of varus. The axis line is drawn from the center of the hip to the center of the ankle. The degree of varus (or valgus) is quantified as follows (▶ Fig. 2.20).

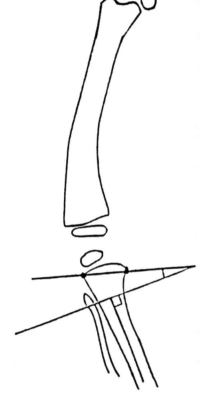

Fig. 2.17 Metaphyseal–diaphyseal angle used to detect tibia vara in very young children. High diagnostic likelihood if angle is greater than 11 to 16 degrees.

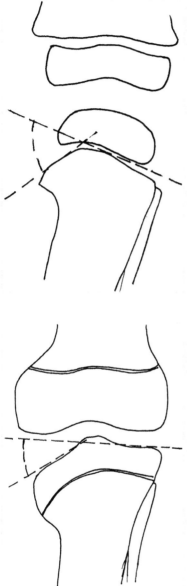

Fig. 2.18 Metaphyseal slope is used to predict the risk of recurrent deformity. Values over 60 degrees are at increased risk.

Fig. 2.19 Medial plateau depression is unique to infantile tibia vara. If greater than 25 degrees, then the medial side may need to be selectively elevated.

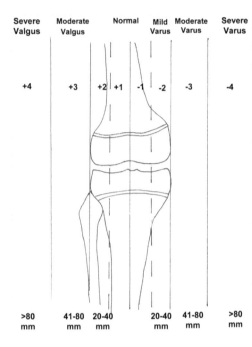

Severe Valgus	Moderate Valgus	Normal		Mild Varus	Moderate Varus	Severe Varus
+4	+3	+2 +1	-1	-2	-3	-4
>80 mm	41-80 mm	20-40 mm		20-40 mm	41-80 mm	>80 mm

Fig. 2.20 Mechanical axis deviation. The location of a straight line between the hip and the ankle is graded in zones as shown.

2.10.2 Differential Diagnosis

1. Rickets: Many types.
2. Achondroplasia.
3. Metaphyseal chondrodysplasia (Schmidt).
4. Trauma or infection of medial physis.
5. Physiologic bowing.
6. Focal fibrocartilaginous dysplasia.

2.10.3 Treatment

1. Infantile:
   a) Observe or brace (day vs. night).
   b) Valgus derotation osteotomy if not better by age 4 or Langenskjold stage 4. Hemiepiphysiodesis is another option up to this stage.
   c) Consider MRI for bar if physis is narrow or medial physeal slope is greater than 60 degrees. If bar is found, resect it or close lateral side of physis.
   d) Consider tibial plateau elevation if medial depression exceeds 25 degrees.

e) Correct femoral valgus deformity if greater than 10 degrees.

f) Equalize leg lengths as needed.

2. Adolescent tibia vara:

a) Correct if deformity exceeds 10 degrees or pain is persistent.

b) Lateral hemiepiphysiodesis is an option if deformity is not severe (mechanical axis deviation 1–2) and patient has two or more years of growth remaining.

c) Osteotomy of proximal tibia and distal femur as appropriate.

d) Equalize leg lengths if discrepancy is greater than 2.5 cm.

Bibliography

1. Feldman MD, Schoenecker PL. Use of the metaphyseal-diaphyseal angle in the evaluation of bowed legs. J Bone Joint Surg Am 1993;75(11):1602–1609

2. Gordon JE, King DJ, Luhmann SJ, Dobbs MB, Schoenecker PL. Femoral deformity in tibia vara. J Bone Joint Surg Am 2006;88(2):380–386

3. Henderson RC, Kemp GJ Jr, Greene WB. Adolescent tibia vara: alternatives for operative treatment. J Bone Joint Surg Am 1992;74(3):342–350

4. McIntosh AL, Hanson CM, Rathjen KE. Treatment of adolescent tibia vara with hemiepiphysiodesis: risk factors for failure. J Bone Joint Surg Am 2009;91(12):2873–2879

5. Park SS, Gordon JE, Luhmann SJ, Dobbs MB, Schoenecker PL. Outcome of hemiepiphyseal stapling for late-onset tibia vara. J Bone Joint Surg Am 2005;87(10):2259–2266

2.11 Other Angular Deformities at the Knee

Angular deformities may occur as a result of trauma or metabolic disorders, or they may be idiopathic or physiologic. If deviation from normal alignment is greater than 10 degrees, correction may be indicated in some cases. Treatment may be done by osteotomy and internal or external fixation or by hemiepiphysiodesis. The goal is to restore a horizontal joint line, physiologic angulation (see Chapter 1, Fig. 1.40), and near-equal limb lengths.

Hemiepiphysiodesis may be the simplest method for growing patients. The theory is shown in ▶ Fig. 2.21. Prerequisites include (1) predictable growth pattern, (2) sufficient growth remaining to correct defect, and (3) limb lengths close to equal.

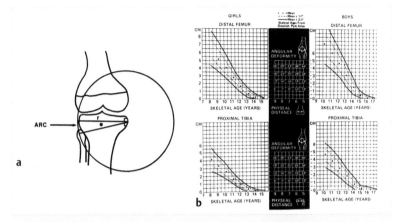

Fig. 2.21 (a) Theory of angular correction by asymmetrical tethering. (b) Angular correction is calculated from metaphyseal width and growth remaining. (Used with permission from Bowen JR, Leahey JL, Zhang ZH, MacEwen GD. Partial epiphysiodesis at the knee to correct angular deformity. Clin Orthop Relat Res 1985;198 (Figs. 2 and 3).)

2.11.1 Planning

1. Locate the site of deformity—distal femur, proximal tibia, or both—and measure its degree.
2. Using the width of the physis and the desired degree of correction, draw a horizontal line on the graph.
3. Draw a dot at the intersection of this horizontal line with the patient's tibial or femoral percentile.
4. A vertical line from this point downward indicates the age at which hemiepiphysiodesis should be performed. If done before puberty, it will indicate the length of time before correction is complete. Allow slight overcorrection before removing plates.

Bibliography

1. Bowen JR, Leahey JL, Zhang ZH, MacEwen GD. Partial epiphysiodesis at the knee to correct angular deformity. Clin Orthop Relat Res 1985;(198):184–190
2. Stevens PM, Klatt JB. Guided growth for pathological physes: radiographic improvement during realignment. J Pediatr Orthop 2008;28(6):632–639

2.12 Patellofemoral Disorders

Patellofemoral disorders are common, especially in adolescence. History should include duration of symptoms, recent changes in activity, and inciting factors.

2.12.1 Physical Examination

1. Patient to indicate location of pain.
2. Check pain on compression of patella.
3. Apprehension test (guarding with lateral pressure).
4. Assess effusion.
5. Note retinacular tightness (reverse tilt).
6. Measure tibial and femoral rotational alignment.
7. Assess ligament and meniscal integrity.
8. Measure valgus.
9. Examine active tracking.
10. Observe gait.

2.12.2 Differential Diagnosis

1. Plica.
2. Saphenous nerve entrapment.
3. Fat pad impingement.
4. Patellar osteochondritis.
5. Iliotibial band syndrome.
6. Patellar malalignment.
7. Patellar subluxation.
8. Arthrosis.

2.12.3 Imaging

Radiographs are not needed on initial evaluation of all cases. However, if the problem is recalcitrant, the following studies may help:

1. Merchant view: A "sunrise" view taken at 30 to 45 degrees of knee flexion (▶ Fig. 2.22a). From this, the sulcus angle can be measured, which should be greater than 17 degrees (▶ Fig. 2.22b).
2. The lateral view will show the Insall ratio, which is the length of tendon divided by the length of patella (▶ Fig. 2.23). The normal value is 1.0, and the upper limit of normal is 1.2.
3. Computed tomography (CT) may be helpful to assess patellar tilt. It should be done in 20 degrees of flexion. Normal tilt is less than + 8 degrees.
4. MRI is an option to assess for osteochondral lesions.
5. Measure tibial tuberal–trochlear groove distance on MRI; Nl < 20 mm.

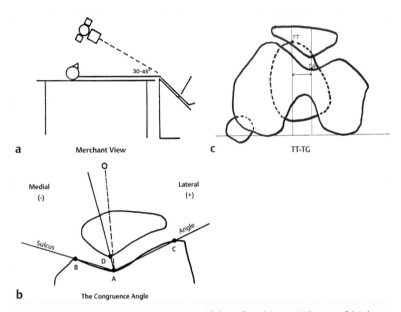

a   Merchant View

c   TT-TG

b   The Congruence Angle

Fig. 2.22 (**a**) Merchant view: a sunrise view with knee flexed 30 to 45 degrees. (**b**) Sulcus angle, B-A-C, is 138 +/- 6 degrees, and congruence angle, D-A-O, should be less than 17 degrees lateral to its bisector. (**c**) Method of measuring Tibial Tubercle to Trochlear Groove distance (TT-TG) on computed tomogram. (Used with permission from Merchant AC, Mercer RL, Jacobsen RH, Cool CR. Roentgenographic analysis of patellofemoral congruence. J Bone Joint Surg Am 1974 Oct;56(7):1391–1396 (Figs. 2 and 5).)

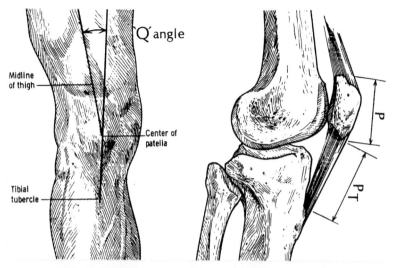

Fig. 2.23 Insall ratio to evaluate the patella alta: length of the tendon is divided by the length of the patella. The patella alto is defined as a ratio of greater than 1.2. P, patella; PT, patella tendon; Q, Q angle. (Used with permission from Insall J, Falvo KA, Wise DW. Chondromalacia patellae: a prospective study. J Bone Joint Surg Am 1976;58(1):2 (Fig. 2).)

2.12.4 Treatment

Treatment of patellofemoral malalignment should start with conservative measures. These may include the following:

1. Stretching of retinaculum, iliotibial band, quadriceps, and hamstrings.
2. Strengthening of quadriceps: Low resistance, high repetition, knee not flexed over 45 degrees.
3. NSAIDs.
4. Orthotics to decrease foot pronation, if present.
5. Elastic brace or patellar taping.
6. In the resistant case, surgical correction may be offered and may include the following:
   a) Lateral release (for tilt).
   b) Tibial tubercle transfer + vastus medialis oblique advancement (for subluxation).
   c) Limited debridement (for severe cartilage surface degeneration).
   d) Optional correction of severe anteversion or torsion.

Bibliography

1. Lubowitz JH, Bernardini BJ, Reid JB III. Current concepts review: comprehensive physical examination for instability of the knee. Am J Sports Med 2008;36(3):577–594

2.13 Discoid Lateral Meniscus

2.13.1 Background and Classification

1. Incidence: About 1%; usually lateral.
2. Classification: Based on the degree of attachment to the tibial plateau:
   a) Wrisberg ligament type: Absent lateral meniscotibial ligaments. Only ligament of Wrisberg present, attaching meniscus to the posterior cruciate ligament. This type is the most anomalous and unstable type.
   b) Complete type: Meniscus covers the entire tibial plateau, but ligaments are intact.
   c) Incomplete type: Stable incomplete discoid meniscus with intact ligaments.

2.13.2 Clinical Signs and Symptoms

1. "Snapping knee," typically before the age of 8 years.
2. A palpable snap and shift of the tibial plateau during movement.
3. Joint pain and swelling occur as the meniscus develops a tear.
4. Feelings of "catching" with knee motion.

2.13.3 Imaging

1. Plain radiographs are indicated initially to rule out any bony anomalies. These may show widening of lateral joint space.
2. MRI shows discoid meniscus and any tears.
3. A true discoid meniscus will appear as a continuous bow-tie appearance on three or more consecutive sagittal plane images. In the coronal plane, the discoid meniscus occupies more than one-third of the joint diameter at the midpoint. False negatives can occur with the unstable (Wrisberg) type of discoid meniscus, which may maintain a relatively semilunar shape.

2.13.4 Treatment

1. If the child is asymptomatic and the discoid meniscus is an incidental finding, then excision is not recommended.

2. Substantial tears of a stable discoid meniscus may require a resection in which the peripheral rim is left intact (meniscoplasty).
3. In cases in which the meniscus is unstable, repair and contouring may be attempted, but a complete meniscectomy may be required.

2.13.5 Prognosis

There is little long-term follow-up data for both untreated discoid menisci and for partial discoid meniscectomy.

Bibliography

1. Dickhaut SC, DeLee JC. The discoid lateral-meniscus syndrome. J Bone Joint Surg Am 1982;64(7):1068–1073
2. Shieh AK, Edmonds EW, Pennock AT. Revision meniscal surgery in children and adolescents: risk factors and mechanisms for failure and subsequent management. Am J Sports Med 2016;44(4):838–843

2.14 Popliteal (Baker) Cyst

2.14.1 Background

1. Popliteal cysts are the most common masses found in the popliteal fossa.
2. These synovial-lined ganglion cysts arise from synovial fluid through communication between the knee joint and the bursa between the semimembranosus and medial gastrocnemius muscles.
3. Located along the medial side of the popliteal fossa, posterior to the medial femoral condyle, between the two tendons.
4. Rarely associated with conditions such as meniscal tears, arthritides, and pigmented villonodular synovitis.
5. Prevalence of popliteal cysts in asymptomatic children is about 2%.

2.14.2 Signs and Symptoms

1. Rarely causes symptoms and is usually an incidental discovery.
2. May wax and wane in size but should not cause limp or disability.
3. However, patients may present with complaints of pain if the cyst ruptures.

2.14.3 Physical Features

Superficial, firm or rubbery, smooth, nontender, slightly mobile, and nonpulsatile mass. Most cysts will transilluminate with a handheld light (▶ Fig. 2.24). If so, imaging is unnecessary.

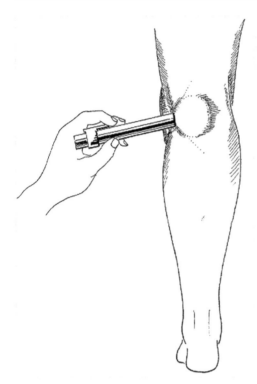

Fig. 2.24 Transillumination of the popliteal cyst. The cyst picks up light more than surrounding tissues.

2.14.4 Imaging

1. Differential diagnosis: Lipomas, xanthomas, vascular tumors, or fibrosarcomas.
2. History and transillumination are the best ways to differentiate.
3. If in doubt, ultrasound can be used to distinguish between fluid-filled cysts and solid tumors. MRI is another option for those rare cases when clinical confirmation is in doubt.

2.14.5 Treatment

Most cysts (85%) disappear without intervention or cause few symptoms (15%). Surgical excision is rarely indicated. Parents should be informed that the cyst may vary in size for a while, but it should eventually regress over the years. Only if the diagnosis is in doubt or if clinical symptoms are persistent should surgery be undertaken.

Bibliography

1. De Greef I, Molenaers G, Fabry G. Popliteal cysts in children: a retrospective study of 62 cases. Acta Orthop Belg 1998;64(2):180–183
2. De Maeseneer M, Debaere C, Desprechins B, Osteaux M. Popliteal cysts in children: prevalence, appearance and associated findings at MR imaging. Pediatr Radiol 1999;29(8):605–609
3. Seil R, Rupp S, Jochum P, Schofer O, Mischo B, Kohn D. Prevalence of popliteal cysts in children. A sonographic study and review of the literature. Arch Orthop Trauma Surg 1999;119(1–2):73–75

2.15 Congenital Dysplasia (Anterolateral Bow/ Pseudarthrosis) of the Tibia

2.15.1 Background and Natural History

1. Congenital dysplasia may be sporadic or associated with neruofibromatosis-1.
2. Etiology is unknown.
3. Anterolateral bowing of the distal tibia resembles genu varum, but the apex is more distal and has an anterior component; it is unilateral only.
4. Bowing often progresses to pseudarthrosis, which is usually very difficult to heal with cast, plate, or electrical stimulation. The distal apex contributes to difficulty with fixation.
5. 1 to 4 cm shortening of the affected side.
6. Clinically no pain until fracture (which produces little pain).

2.15.2 Imaging (▶ Fig. 2.25)

1. Narrowing of tibia at bow.
2. Narrowing or scalloping of medullary canal.
3. Tapering of bone ends.
4. May be associated with fibular bowing or pseudarthrosis.

2.15.3 Treatment

1. Protect with brace before fracture.
2. Fibular strut if fracture is imminent.
3. If fractured, options include long intramedullary (Williams) rod ± rhBMP-2, Ilizarov treatment, free vascularized fibula, or combinations.
4. Separate treatment for limb-length inequality and valgus ankle may be required.

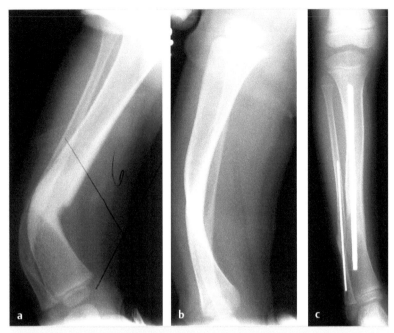

Fig. 2.25 Anteroposterior (**a**) and lateral (**b**) radiographs of a 3-year-old with neurofibromatosis-1 and congenital tibial dysplasia before the fracture. (**c**) Two years after the fracture and rodding.

Bibliography

1. Dobbs MB, Rich MM, Gordon JE, Szymanski DA, Schoenecker PL. Use of an intramedullary rod for treatment of congenital pseudarthrosis of the tibia. A long-term follow-up study. J Bone Joint Surg Am 2004;86-A(6):1186–1197
2. Dobbs MB, Rich MM, Gordon JE, Szymanski DA, Schoenecker PL. Use of an intramedullary rod for the treatment of congenital pseudarthrosis of the tibia. Surgical technique. J Bone Joint Surg Am 2005; 87(Pt 1, Suppl 1):33–40
3. Ofluoglu O, Davidson RS, Dormans JP. Prophylactic bypass grafting and long-term bracing in the management of anterolateral bowing of the tibia and neurofibromatosis-1. J Bone Joint Surg Am 2008;90(10):2126–2134
4. Richards BS, Oetgen ME, Johnston CE. The use of rhBMP-2 for the treatment of congenital pseudarthrosis of the tibia: a case series. J Bone Joint Surg Am 2010;92(1):177–185

2.16 Posteromedial Bow of Tibia
2.16.1 Background and Natural History

1. Present at birth; etiology unknown; not a prior fracture.
2. Bowing resolves with time and growth over 5 to 10 years.
3. No increased risk of fracture.
4. Shortening proportionate throughout growth; mean 2 to 5 cm at maturity.

2.16.2 Clinical and Imaging (▶ Fig. 2.26)

1. Foot appears dorsiflexed and in valgus; limited plantar flexion.
2. Leg slightly short at birth.
3. Tibia and fibula have posteromedial bow of distal third with sclerotic cortices.

2.16.3 Treatment

1. Observation with or without stretching and orthosis for foot support.
2. Osteotomy rarely necessary for bowing.
3. Leg-length equalization as indicated, with lift and surgery near maturity.

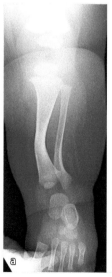 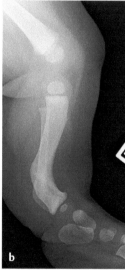

Fig. 2.26 (a,b) Posteromedial bowing of the tibia and fibula in a 1-year-old.

Bibliography

1. Pappas AM. Congenital posteromedial bowing of the tibia and fibula. J Pediatr Orthop 1984;4(5):525–531
2. Shah HH, Doddabasappa SN, Joseph B. Congenital posteromedial bowing of the tibia: a retrospective analysis of growth abnormalities in the leg. J Pediatr Orthop B 2009;18(3):120–128

2.17 Clubfoot

Talipes equinovarus may be unilateral or bilateral with equal frequency. Although most cases are idiopathic, other causes or associations should be considered:
1. Neurogenic: Spinal dysraphism, tethered cord, arthrogryposis.
2. Connective tissue disorders: Loeys–Dietz syndrome, Larsen syndrome, diastrophic dwarfism, spondyloepiphyseal dysplasia.
3. Mechanical: Oligohydramnios, congenital constriction bands.
4. Syndromes: Freeman–Sheldon, Pierre-Robin, tibial hemimelia, Mobius.

2.17.1 Physical Findings

A variable number of these findings may be present:
1. Medial or posterior crease.
2. Curved lateral border.
3. Calf atrophy.
4. Cavus.
5. Equinus.
6. Forefoot adduction and supination.

The foot may be given a DiMeglio score from 1 to 20 if each positive finding is awarded 1 point (▶ Table 2.2).

2.17.2 Imaging

Radiographs are useful if surgery is indicated or in postsurgical follow-up. AP and lateral films should be taken with the foot as plantigrade as possible. Normal values for AP and lateral talocalcaneal angles are given in Chapter 1 (Fig. 1.46 and Fig. 1.47). Equinovarus correlates with increasing parallelism of the talus and calcaneus. Cuboid can be neutral or subluxated medially.

Table 2.2 The DiMeglio Clubfoot Scoring System (very severe = 16–20, severe = 11–16, moderate = 6–10, postural = 1–5)

Parameter	Points				
	4 (degrees)	3 (degrees)	2 (degrees)	1 (degrees)	0 (degrees)
Equinus	45–90	20–45	20–0	0–20 DF	>+20 DF
Varus	45–90	20–45	20–0	0–20 DF	>20 val
Supination	45–90	20–45	20–0	0–20 pro	>20 pro
Adductus	45–90	20–45	20–0	0–20	>20 abd
Posterior crease				Yes	No
Medial crease				Yes	No
Cavus				Yes	No
Abnl muscle fcn				Yes	No

Abbreviations: Abd, abduction; Abnl, abnormal; DF, dorsiflexion; fcn, function; pro, pronation; val, valgus.

2.17.3 Treatment

1. Serial manipulation and long-leg cast treatment (Ponseti method): This treatment produces the most normal foot growth and mobility; it is described in greater detail in Chapter 9. Sequence of correction:
   a) Dorsiflexion/supination of first ray.
   b) Counterpressure on dorsolateral aspect of talus.
   c) Progressive external rotation and dorsiflexion of hindfoot.
   d) Achilles tenotomy if correction of hindfoot equinus is not complete after correction of other components.
   e) Maintaining correction after cast removal with *foot abduction orthosis*. This is a pair of straight- or reverse-last shoes attached to a bar with the feet externally rotated 60 degrees.
   f) Foot abduction orthosis is worn full time for 2 months, then nightly for 3 to 5 years.
   g) Relapses are salvaged by repeat cast program.
   h) Feet with late recurrence are treated by Achilles tendon lengthening and transfer of the anterior tibialis to the third cuneiform.
2. Operative correction, for severe relapses and syndromes, may include the following:
   a) Lengthening of heel cord and posterior tibialis.
   b) Posteromedial capsulotomies.
   c) Complete subtalar release.
   d) Calcaneocuboid release.
   e) Lateral column shortening.

Bibliography

1. DiMeglio A, Bensahel H, Souchet P, Mazeau P, Bonnet F. Classification of clubfoot. J Pediatr Orthop B 1995;4(2):129–136
2. Dobbs MB, Rudzki JR, Purcell DB, Walton T, Porter KR, Gurnett CA. Factors predictive of outcome after use of the Ponseti method for the treatment of idiopathic clubfeet. J Bone Joint Surg Am 2004;86-A(1):22–27
3. Holt JB, Oji DE, Yack HJ, Morcuende JA. Long-term results of tibialis anterior tendon transfer for relapsed idiopathic clubfoot treated with the Ponseti method: a follow-up of thirty-seven to fifty-five years. J Bone Joint Surg Am 2015;97(1):47–55
4. Hosseinzadeh P, Kelly DM, Zionts LE. Management of the relapsed clubfoot following treatment using the Ponseti method. J Am Acad Orthop Surg 2017;25(3):195–203
5. Ponseti IV. The Ponseti technique for correction of congenital clubfoot. J Bone Joint Surg Am 2002;84-A(10):1889–1890, author reply 1890–1891

2.18 Tarsal Coalition

Tarsal coalition is a fibrous, cartilaginous, or bony connection of two or more tarsal bones. It is present in about 3% of the population and is bilateral in half of these. Calcaneonavicular (CN) and talocalcaneal (TC) bars are equally common.

2.18.1 Signs and Symptoms

1. Foot or ankle pain and stiffness occurs at about age 8 to 12 years for CN bar, 12 to 16 for TC bar.
2. Limitation of subtalar movement is greater with TC coalition.
3. Pes planus: Variable.
4. Peroneal guarding or "spasm."

2.18.2 Imaging

1. Oblique view of the midfoot is diagnostic for a CN bar with narrowing, irregularity, or fusion of the space between the two bones (▶ Fig. 2.27a).
2. Lateral view shows pointed projection of calcaneus or "anteater nose" in CN coalition.
3. Harris view shows obliquity and sclerosis of sustentaculum in TC coalition and may show fusion across the middle facet.

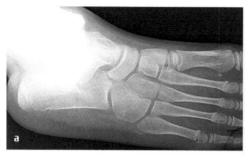

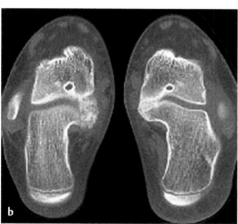

Fig. 2.27 (a) Oblique view of the midfoot is diagnostic for the calcaneonavicular bar with narrowing, irregularity, or fusion of the space between the two bones. (b) Computed tomography is the definitive study for a talocalcaneal coalition. The plane of the tomograms should be the coronal plane of the foot with the knees flexed and the sole flat on the gantry. Reconstructions in all planes should be viewed.

4. CT is the definitive study for a TC coalition. The plane of the tomograms should be the coronal plane of the foot with the knees flexed and the sole flat on the gantry. Reconstructions in all planes should be viewed (▶ Fig. 2.27b).
5. CN and TC coalitions may coexist.

2.18.3 Treatment

1. If discovered incidentally and asymptomatic, observe.
2. Arch support.
3. Walking cast for 3 to 6 weeks.
4. Bar resection if conservative treatment (1-3 above) fails for a TC bar less than 50% and no degenerative changes or a CN bar of any size.
5. Arthrodesis.

Bibliography

1. Lemley F, Berlet G, Hill K, Philbin T, Isaac B, Lee T. Current concepts review: tarsal coalition. Foot Ankle Int 2006;27(12):1163–1169

2.19 Flatfoot

2.19.1 Background and Definition

1. Etiology is a combination of factors, including connective tissue properties, muscle tone, and genetics.
2. Achilles contracture increases eversion as compensatory dorsiflexion occurs through the subtalar joint.

2.19.2 Signs and Symptoms

1. Usually asymptomatic.
2. Severe pressure on plantar-medial surface may cause pain.
3. The natural history is generally benign in all but the most pronounced cases.

2.19.3 Physical Features and Examination

1. Examine elbows, wrists, and knees for evidence of ligamentous laxity.
2. Determine range of hindfoot and forefoot motion to classify as flexible or rigid.
3. Measure ankle dorsiflexion.
4. Observe patient standing on toes, checking for reappearance of the arch as an indicator of structural integrity of the foot during push-off ("heel-rise test").
5. Inspect skin of sole for signs of pressure concentration over navicular and talar head.

2.19.4 Differential Diagnosis

1. Connective tissue disorders: Marfan, Ehlers–Danlos, osteogenesis imperfecta.
2. Neurologic disorders: Spinal dysraphism, diplegia.
3. Tarsal coalition: Fibrous or bony.
4. Congenital malformation: Fibular hemimelia, vertical talus.
5. Accessory navicular.

2.19.5 Treatment

1. Observation if asymptomatic.
2. Soft arch support if symptoms are severe.
3. Surgical reconstruction if symptoms are unresponsive, with structural weakness and pressure concentration.

Bibliography

1. Bauer K, Mosca VS, Zionts LE. What's new in pediatric flatfoot? J Pediatr Orthop 2016;36(8):865–869
2. Kasser JR. The pediatric foot. In: Morrissy RT, Weinstein SL, eds. Lovell and Winter's Pediatric Orthopaedics. 6th ed. Philadelphia, PA: Lippincott Williams & Wilkins; 2008:1257–1329

2.20 Calcaneovalgus Foot

Positional deformity in newborns. The foot is dorsiflexed at the ankle and in valgus.

2.20.1 Physical Features

Passively, the foot may be plantarflexed to neutral or below, but it does not have a full range of normal plantarflexion. There is no deformity of the tibia.

2.20.2 Imaging

Radiographs are not indicated in the typical case because physical examination is diagnostic. If radiographs are obtained, then they show no bony abnormalities other than the dorsiflexed position. This differentiates it from posteromedial bow of the tibia.

2.20.3 Treatment

No treatment is necessary. Deformity improves with time. No casting, bracing, or splinting is necessary.

2.20.4 Prognosis

Spontaneous resolution is the rule.

Bibliography

1. Kasser JR. The pediatric foot. In: Morrissy RT, Weinstein SL, eds. Lovell and Winter's Pediatric Orthopaedics. 6th ed. Philadelphia, PA: Lippincott Williams & Wilkins; 2008:1257–1329

2.21 Congenital Vertical Talus

Essential feature is a dorsolateral dislocation of the talonavicular joint with associated contractures.

2.21.1 Etiology

1. Idiopathic.
2. Myelomeningocele.
3. Arthrogryposis.
4. Larsen syndrome.

2.21.2 Physical Findings

1. Reversal of arch with plantar convexity, "rocker bottom."
2. Forefoot is dorsiflexed and everted; hindfoot is plantar flexed.
3. Normal arch is not reproducible.
4. Crease in sinus tarsi.

2.21.3 Imaging

1. Talus is almost "vertical" and is in line with tibia.
2. Talar axis does not line up with first metatarsal.
3. Diagnostic test: Talus and first metatarsal still do not line up with stress plantarflexion lateral film of foot (▶ Fig. 2.28).

2.21.4 Treatment

1. Plantarflexion casting (into clubfoot position).
2. Percutaneous pinning of talonavicular joint.
3. Open reduction via dorsal or plantar approach, with tendon lengthening.
4. Subtalar fusion if valgus persists.

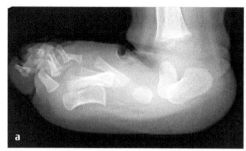

Fig. 2.28 (a,b) Diagnostic test for congenital vertical talus. The talus and first metatarsal still do not line up with stress plantarflexion lateral film of foot.

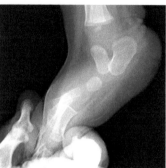

Bibliography

1. Seimon LP. Surgical correction of congenital vertical talus under the age of 2 years. J Pediatr Orthop 1987;7(4):405–411
2. Yang JS, Dobbs MB. Treatment of congenital vertical talus: comparison of minimally invasive and extensive soft-tissue release procedures at minimum five-year follow-up. J Bone Joint Surg Am 2015;97(16):1354–1365

2.22 Hallux Valgus

2.22.1 Background and Definitions

1. First metatarsophalangeal (MTP) angle is greater than 15 degrees.
2. Onset before age 10 is termed *juvenile hallux valgus.*
3. Onset between age 10 and 18 is termed *adolescent hallux valgus.*
4. Positive family history and ligamentous laxity are common.

2.22.2 Clinical Features

1. Asymptomatic or pain over medial prominence.
2. Tightness of Achilles tendon may be present.
3. Pes planus is usually present.
4. Range of toe movement should be measured.

2.22.3 Imaging

1. Standing AP and lateral radiographs are needed.
2. MTP angle greater than 15 degrees is hallux valgus (▶ Fig. 2.29).

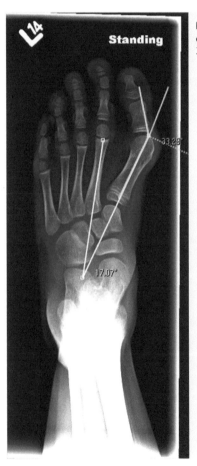

Fig. 2.29 Intermetatarsal angle of 17 degrees and metatarsophalangeal angle of 33 degrees.

3. An intermetatarsal angle (between the first and second metatarsals) greater than 10 degrees indicates metatarsus primus varus (MPV).
4. The distal metatarsal articular angle (DMAA) is formed between the shaft of the first metatarsal and the line perpendicular to the articular surface of the MTP joint. The DMAA is expected to increase in juvenile or adolescent hallux vagus.
5. MTP joint congruity, relative lengths of the metatarsals, metatarsocuneiform orientation, proximal phalangeal articular angle, and lesser metatarsal orientation should also be assessed.

2.22.4 Treatment

1. Conservative treatment is the mainstay: Shoes should be made of soft material and a low heel. Arch supports may help with pronation.
2. Surgery is indicated only if there is significant pain despite conservative treatment.
3. MPV in adolescent: Lateral hemiepiphysiodesis of first metatarsal base.
4. Deformity of interphalangeal joint (hallux valgus interphalangeus): Osteotomy of proximal phalanx.
5. MTP less than 25 degrees: Soft-tissue reconstruction.
6. MTP greater than 25 degrees in mature, symptomatic patient: Correct MPV and reorient joint.
7. Address significant hindfoot valgus with osteotomies.
8. Arthrodesis of the MTP joint is the most reliable way to correct hallux valgus in cerebral palsy.

2.22.5 Complications

Stiffness of the MTP joint, persistent pain, AVN of the metatarsal head, and a high rate of recurrence.

Bibliography

1. Aronson J, Nguyen LL, Aronson EA. Early results of the modified Peterson bunion procedure for adolescent hallux valgus. J Pediatr Orthop 2001;21 (1):65–69
2. Davids JR, McBrayer D, Blackhurst DW. Juvenile hallux valgus deformity: surgical management by lateral hemiepiphyseodesis of the great toe metatarsal. J Pediatr Orthop 2007;27(7):826–830
3. Groiso JA. Juvenile hallux valgus. A conservative approach to treatment. J Bone Joint Surg Am 1992;74(9):1367–1374

2.23 Toe Walking

2.23.1 Background

1. Common in toddlers.
2. Commonly caused by shortened Achilles tendon.
3. Some eventually adopt normal walking with growth.
4. Persistent toe walking beyond 3 years of age should prompt examination for underlying neuromuscular problems.
5. However, most children have, by exclusion, *idiopathic toe walking.*
6. Many patients have a positive family history.
7. May be associated with autism, language disorders.

2.23.2 Signs and Symptoms

1. Painless.
2. Occasionally frequent falling.

2.23.3 Physical Examination

1. Examine with the child in shorts.
2. Assess for ataxia, muscle weakness, Gowers sign.
3. Range of ankle dorsiflexion should be noted, with the knee both flexed and extended.
4. Look for calf pseudohypertrophy.
5. Hamstrings and adductors should be checked for tightness.

2.23.4 Differential Diagnosis

1. Cerebral palsy.
2. Muscular dystrophy.
3. Tethered cord syndrome.
4. Charcot–Marie–Tooth disease.
5. Arthrogryposis.
6. Friedreich ataxia.

2.23.5 Treatment

1. Physical therapy.
2. Casting: Increased ankle dorsiflexion can be achieved by stretching and serial casting. The cast should be changed weekly until the desired ankle range of motion is obtained. After casts are off, continue stretching.
3. Achilles tendon lengthening, percutaneous or open.

Bibliography

1. Engström P, Tedroff K. The prevalence and course of idiopathic toe-walking in 5-year-old children. Pediatrics 2012;130(2):279–284
2. Kalen V, Adler N, Bleck EE. Electromyography of idiopathic toe walking. J Pediatr Orthop 1986;6(1):31–33

2.24 Macrodactyly

2.24.1 Background

1. Macrodactyly is overgrowth of one or several adjacent digits or rays of a hand or foot.
2. It is present at birth, although some cases worsen disproportionately.
3. Growth of the enlarged digits ceases when the patient reaches skeletal maturity.

2.24.2 Classification

1. Incidence is less than 1:10,000.
2. Most cases are idiopathic; others are associated with Klippel–Trenaunay–Weber syndrome, neurofibromatosis-1 (NF-1), or Proteus syndrome.
3. Usually unilateral.
4. Etiology unknown.
5. No genetic risk if not NF-1.

2.24.3 Signs and Symptoms

1. Painless in child; premature arthritis in adult.
2. Difficulty with shoe wear.
3. Impaired push-off (foot) or clumsiness (hand).

2.24.4 Physical Features (▶ Fig. 2.30)

1. Enlargement is greater distally than proximally. The nail is especially enlarged. All tissues are affected.
2. Tissues on the plantar or palmar surface of the digit are more enlarged than those on the dorsal side, causing the digit to become hyperextended (dorsiflexed).
3. Central digits are more commonly involved than border digits.
4. Syndactyl may coexist.
5. Metatarsals and carpals are rarely significantly enlarged.

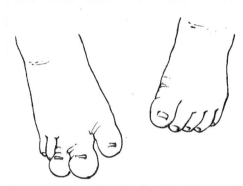

Fig. 2.30 Physical features of macrodactyly.

6. If two digits are involved, they grow away from each other.
7. Rarely enlargement is disproportionate.
8. Skin may display hemangioma.
9. Range of interphalangeal motion is decreased.

2.24.5 Tests

Genetic testing is available for Proteus syndrome and NF if these are suspected.

2.24.6 Imaging

1. Plain films should be made to help assess and document the extent of overgrowth and the segments involved.
2. Skeletal maturity is often advanced in the enlarged rays.
3. MRI is rarely necessary.

2.24.7 Differential Diagnosis

1. Hemihypertrophy, in which all segments of a limb are uniformly overgrown.
2. Acrodactyly, in which overgrowth of all digits is greatest distally.
3. Growth hormone excess: Acromegaly.

2.24.8 Treatment

1. Shoe modification if needed.
2. Surgery:
   a) Resection of the most enlarged ray, if the width of the hand or foot is greatly increased.

   b) Phalangectomy may make the length more even if the width is not a problem (if nail loss is acceptable).

   c) Epiphysiodesis (closure of the growth plates); the correction occurs more gradually with time.

3. Debulking of fat may improve the appearance, especially of the plantar fat hypertrophy.

4. Discretion advised in staging multiple procedures to avoid tissue ischemia.

Bibliography

1. Akinci M, Ay S, Erçetin O. Surgical treatment of macrodactyly in older children and adults. J Hand Surg Am 2004;29(6):1010–1019
2. Barsky AJ. Macrodactyly. J Bone Joint Surg Am 1967;49(7):1255–1266
3. Dennyson WG, Bear JN, Bhoola KD. Macrodactyly in the foot. J Bone Joint Surg Br 1977;59(3):355–359
4. Kim J, Park JW, Hong SW, Jeong JY, Gong HS, Baek GH. Ray amputation for the treatment of foot macrodactyly in children. Bone Joint J 2015;97-B (10):1364–1369
5. Waters PM, Gillespie BT. Ray resection for progressive macrodactyly of the hand: surgical technique and illustrative cases. J Hand Surg Am 2016;41(8): e251–e256

3 Disorders of Spinal Growth and Development

Paul D. Sponseller

3.1 Torticollis

Malposition of the head and neck with lateral flexion to one side and rotation to the contralateral side. The child holds the ear closer to one shoulder and the chin closer to the other.

3.1.1 Differential Diagnosis

1. Muscular torticollis resulting from contracture of sternocleidomastoid.
2. Atlantoaxial rotatory instability.
3. Congenital bony malformation of upper cervical spine.
4. Reflux response (Sandifer syndrome).
5. Ocular or auditory abnormality.
6. Brainstem abnormality or tumor.

3.1.2 Physical Examination and Findings

1. Measure range of motion to each side.
2. Thorough neurologic examination.
3. Palpate for sternocleidomastoid contracture (typically tight on the side of the lower ear).
4. Examine eye movements and hearing.
5. Plagiocephaly is a sign of early onset, longer duration.

3.1.3 Imaging

1. Plain films centered on upper cervical spine:
    a) Usually difficult to interpret because of rotation.
    b) Include anteroposterior open mouth view if possible.
2. CT with reconstructions usually necessary when treatment is needed.
3. MRI if neurologic abnormality is suspected or if surgery is planned.

3.1.4 Treatment

1. Muscular torticollis: Stretching, possible lengthening.
2. Atlantoaxial rotatory instability: Stretching if duration less than 1 week; traction if 1 to 3 weeks; fusion if over 1 to 3 months.

3.2 Idiopathic Scoliosis

Idiopathic scoliosis is the most common pediatric spinal deformity. It is transmitted as an autosomal dominant condition with incomplete penetrance. The initial evaluation should rule out other causes and determine maturity, curve size, type, and appropriate treatment.

1. Infantile scoliosis (onset 0–3 years): obtain MRI.
2. Juvenile scoliosis (onset 4–9 years): obtain MRI.
3. Adolescent scoliosis (onset > 9 years): routine MRI not indicated.

3.2.1 History

1. How curve was discovered.
2. Presence or absence of significant pain.
3. Family history.
4. Menarchal status.
5. Medical and surgical history.

3.2.2 Physical Findings and Examination

1. Record height and weight.
2. Assess trunk and extremities for cutaneous lesions, congenital malformation, connective tissue disorder, or atrophy.
3. Measure pelvic height for inequality of lower-limb length.
4. Neurologic examination:
   a) Strength, reflexes all extremities.
   b) Abdominal reflex testing.
5. Estimate physical maturity (breast appearance, facial or axillary hair).
6. Assess curve:
   a) Shoulder elevation.
   b) Trunk balance C1 through S1, coronal and sagittal.
   c) Curve level.
   d) Intrinsic pelvic deformity.
   e) Kyphosis and lordosis.

3.2.3 Differential Diagnosis (in Absence of Overt Vertebral Malformations)

1. Genetic or connective tissue:
   a) Marfan syndrome, Loeys–Dietz syndrome.
   b) Ehlers–Danlos syndrome.
   c) Neurofibromatosis.

109

d) Prader–Willi syndrome.

e) Stickler syndrome.

f) Many others.

2. Neurologic:

a) Syringomyelia.

b) Brainstem or cord tumor.

c) Friedreich ataxia.

d) Charcot–Marie–Tooth disease.

e) Polio

f) Thoracic-level paralysis or dyscoordination of any cause.

3. Neoplastic and other:

a) Tethered cord/occult dysraphism.

b) Osteoid osteoma.

c) Osteoblastoma.

d) Postradiation.

e) Spinal cord tumor.

3.2.4 Scoliosis Screening: Forward-Bend Test (▶ Fig. 3.1)

1. Patient stands with feet together, knees straight, palms together. Check shoulders and pelvis for obliquity, and equalize leg lengths with blocks if necessary. Observe sagittal profile for focal kyphosis.

2. Have patient bend slowly all the way over.

3. Check thoracic spine.

4. Check lumbar spine.

5. Scoliometer measurement of trunk asymmetry (▶ Fig. 3.2). It measures the angle of trunk rotation. This is roughly coordinated with the Cobb angle. A scoliometer reading of 5 or less is 99% sensitive and 97% specific for curves less than a 20-degree Cobb angle. The mean Cobb measurement for curves 5 degrees by scoliometer is 11 degrees. A scoliometer reading of 7 or less is 88% sensitive and 86% specific for curves less than 25 degrees with a mean Cobb of 20 degrees. The scoliometer is adequately sensitive for scoliosis screening: 95% of curves greater than 20 degrees measure 7 degrees or more on the scoliometer. Obesity may mask significant scoliosis, however.

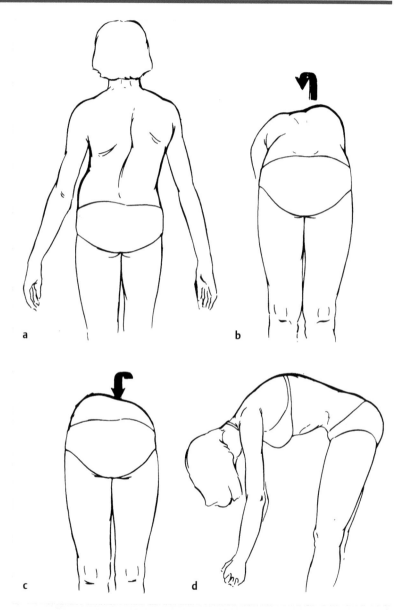

Fig. 3.1 (a-d) Forward-bending test for spinal deformity.

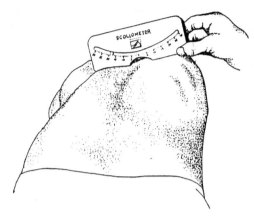

Fig. 3.2 Technique of scoliometer measurement. (Used with permission from Bunnell WP. An objective criterion for scoliosis screening. J Bone Joint Surg Am 1984;66(9):1383 (Fig. 3).)

Bibliography

1. Bunnell WP. Outcome of spinal screening. Spine 1993;18(12):1572–1580
2. Margalit A, McKean G, Constantine A, Thompson CB, Lee RJ, Sponseller PD. Body mass hides the curve: thoracic scoliometer readings vary by body mass index value. J Pediatr Orthop 2017;37(4):e255–e260

3.2.5 Imaging

1. A radiograph should be made if the physical examination indicates that a curve may require treatment. Posteroanterior technique minimizes dose to gonads and breast but gives slightly less detail. A lateral film should be ordered only if needed for evaluation of pain or sagittal deformity. The EOS slot-scanner provides the lowest dose.
2. Look for other anomalies, such as congenital malformation, vertebral erosion, or pedicle widening or thinning. The curve magnitude may be described by the Cobb measurement (▶ Fig. 3.3) and the direction of convexity and levels involved. The interobserver measurement error (Cobb) is around 5 degrees for idiopathic scoliosis and greater than 10 degrees for congenital scoliosis. Skeletal maturity may be roughly estimated by the Risser sign but should be correlated with physical examination (Tanner) and bone age if needed (see Chapter 1 [Fig. 1.12 and Fig. 1.18]).
3. Rotation in the adolescent may be estimated by the method of Nash and Moe (▶ Fig. 3.4) or by CT or the Perdriolle method.

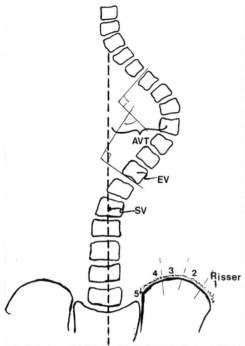

Fig. 3.3 Cobb method of measurement. The angle between the upper and lower end vertebrae (EV) in the curve. Risser sign reflects maturation of the ilium. Grade 5 is fused epiphyses. It has a rough correlation with skeletal age and helps predict the end of skeletal growth. It should not be used in isolation. The stable vertebra is the lowest vertebra bisected by a vertical line from the center of the sacrum. The apical vertebral translation is measured with respect to the central sacral line.

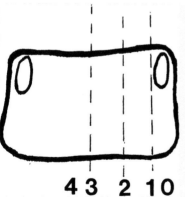

Fig. 3.4 Rotation may be estimated by the method of Nash and Moe according to the location of the pedicle on the convex side.

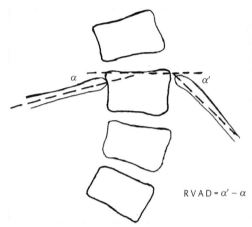

Fig. 3.5 Rotation in infantile curves may be estimated by the rib vertebra angle difference (RVAD) of Mehta. The difference is between the angles formed by the two ribs versus the endplate of the apical vertebra.

$$RVAD = \alpha' - \alpha$$

4. Rotation may be estimated in the infantile or juvenile patient using the rib vertebra angle difference (RVAD) of Mehta (▶ Fig. 3.5).
5. Curve types are named for the level of the apex:
   a) Thoracolumbar curves have an apex at or between T12 and L1.
      1. Thoracic curves have an apex above this.
      2. Lumbar curves have an apex below this.
   b) The Lenke classification of curve types is more comprehensive and incorporates sagittal characteristics (▶ Fig. 3.6).
      1. Main thoracic.
      2. Double thoracic.
      3. Double major.
      4. Triple major.
      5. Thoracolumbar/lumbar.
      6. Thoracolumbar/lumbar: Main thoracic.

3.2.6 Treatment Guidelines

These represent the mainstream of thought, but each case must be managed individually (▶ Fig. 3.7).
1. Infantile scoliosis:
   a) If patient is younger than 1 year or curve is less than about 25 degrees, observe with follow-up in about 4 months.
   b) Obtain MRI if curve is greater than about 25 degrees.
   c) If RVAD is greater than 20 degrees or curve is greater than 35 degrees, consider Mehta casting followed by bracing in younger patients.
   d) If curve progresses to greater than about 60 to 70 degrees, consider growing rods.

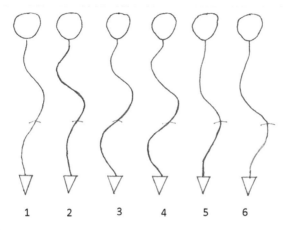

1   2   3   4   5   6

Curve type

Type	Proximal thoracic	Main thoracic	Thoracolumbar / lumbar	Curve type
1	Non-structural	Structural (major*)	Non-structural	Main thoracic (MT)
2	Structural	Structural (major*)	Non-structural	Double thoracic (DT)
3	Non-structural	Structural (major*)	Structural	Double major* (DM)
4	Structural	Structural (major*)	Structural	Triple major* (TM)
5	Non-structural	Non-structural	Structural (major*)	Thoracolumbar / lumbar (TL/L)
6	Non-structural	Structural	Structural (major*)	Thoracolumbar / lumbar (TL/L) Main thoracic (TL/L-MT)

*Major = Largest curve identified by Cobb Measurement always structural
Structural curve = does not bend to 25 degrees or includes T2-5 or T10-L2 kyphosis 20 degrees

Modifiers

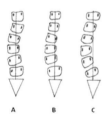

A   B   C

Lumbar Spine Modifier	CSVL to Lumbar Apex	Thoracic Sagittal Profile T5-T12
A	CSVL Between Pedicles	- (Hypo) < 10°
B	CSVL Touches Apical Body (ies)	N (Normal) 10° - 40°
C	CSVL Completely Medial	+ (Hyper) > 40°

Lumbar modifiers: A: Center sacral vertical line (CSVL) falls between pedicles of apical vertebra; B: CSVL touches pedicles of apical vertebra; C: CSVL does not touch apical vertebra

Thoracic sagittal modifier for T5-12: + (> 40°), N (10-40°), - (<10°)

Fig. 3.6 Lenke classification of curve types.

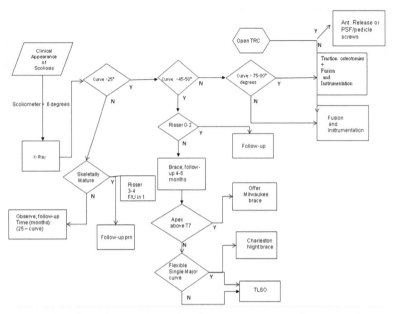

Fig. 3.7 Idiopathic scoliosis treatment algorithm. PSF, posterior spine fusion; TLSO, brace (thoracolumbosacral orthosis); TRC, triradiate cartilage.

2. Juvenile scoliosis:
   a) If curve is greater than 25 degrees, order MRI.
   b) If curve is greater than 25 degrees, consider full-time brace.
   c) If curve progresses beyond 50 to 60 degrees, consider growing rods (or tethering) if the patient is younger than 9 years or definitive fusion if the patient is 10 years or older.
3. Adolescent scoliosis:
   a) Curve over 25 degrees, Risser 0 to 2: Brace full-time (part-time braces less effective for double curves or those over 35 degrees).
   b) Risser 3 + : Observe or night-brace for relevant patterns.
   c) Discontinue brace when Risser is 5 and height gain is less than 1 cm in 6 months.
   d) Curve greater than 50 to 60 degrees: Discuss surgery.

3.3 Back Pain in Children

Although disabling back pain in children is rare, back pain of some degree is experienced by over 30% of children. History should include the following:
1. Precipitating factors.
2. Duration.
3. Severity (1–10).
4. Interference with school, play, or sports.

3.3.1 Physical Examination

1. Neurologic examination.
2. Spinal range of motion.
3. Location of pain.
4. Straight leg raising.

3.3.2 Differential Diagnosis

1. Developmental:
    a) Spondylolysis (most common).
    b) Scheuermann kyphosis (second most common).
    c) Tethered cord.
2. Traumatic:
    a) Herniated nucleus pulposus or endplate.
    b) Musculoligamentous strain.
    c) Fracture.
3. Infectious:
    a) Discitis.
    b) Osteomyelitis.
    c) Tuberculosis.
    d) Sacroiliac joint infection.
4. Tumor:
    a) Benign bony neoplasm:
        1. Osteoid osteoma.
        2. Osteoblastoma.
        3. Aneurysmal bone cyst.
        4. Eosinophilic granuloma.
    b) Malignant bony neoplasm:
        1. Ewing sarcoma.
        2. Osteogenic sarcoma.
        3. Leukemia.
    c) Neoplasm: Neural:
        1. Glioma.

   2. Epidermoid.

   3. Neuroblastoma.

5. Inflammatory:

   a) Ankylosing spondylitis.

   b) Enteropathic arthritis.

6. Extraspinal:

   a) Neural.

   b) Intestinal/pancreatic/renal.

   c) Vascular.

   d) Psychological.

3.3.3 Warning Signs of a Serious Underlying Disorder

1. Neurologic abnormality.
2. Repeated interference with function (school, play, sports).
3. Prolonged stiffness.
4. Fever.

3.3.4 Imaging and Treatment

If warning signs are present, then aggressive workup including plain radiographs or MRI is indicated. If not, close follow-up with appropriate activity modification followed by an exercise program for abdominal and extensor muscles may be used at first. Most patients improve with these. Further tests and treatment should then be undertaken if needed.

Bibliography

1. MacDonald J, Stuart E, Rodenberg R. Musculoskeletal low back pain in school-aged children: a review. JAMA Pediatr 2017;171(3):280–287

3.4 Congenital Scoliosis

1. Definition: Scoliosis that is due to primary vertebral malformation.
2. Types:

   a) Failure of segmentation (Bar): Most deforming (progression 5 degrees or more/year).

   b) Failure of formation (hemivertebra):

     1. Segmented (normal growth plates on either side): Progress up to 2 degrees per year.

     2. Semisegmented.

     3. Unsegmented (nonprogressive).

3. Progression is greatest in first 2 years of life or in adolescent growth spurt.

3.4.1 Associated Findings

1. Spinal dysraphism.
2. VATER (vertebral defects [imperforate] anus, tracheoesophageal [fistula], radial and renal [dysplasia]) or VACTERLS association (vertebral anal, cardiac, tracheal, esophageal, renal, limb, single umbilical artery) malformations.
3. Goldenhar syndrome (oculoauriculovertebral dysplasia).
4. Arthrogryposis.
5. Multiple pterygium syndrome.
6. Skeletal dysplasia.
7. Klippel–Feil syndrome.
8. Sprengel anomaly (congenital scapular elevation).

3.4.2 Imaging

1. Compare films from infancy.
2. Coned anteroposterior and oblique films.
3. Cardiac auscultation.
4. Renal ultrasound or intravenous pyelogram.
5. MRI if there is neurologic asymmetry or if surgery is planned.
6. *Note*: Measurement error is greater than that in idiopathic scoliosis: 10 to 19 degrees.

3.4.3 Treatment

1. Bracing has little or no value.
2. Document progression with films taken in same position every 6 to 12 months.
3. If progressive:
   a) Acceptable deformity: Fuse in situ (anterior and posterior if well-formed vertebral body).
   b) Unacceptable deformity:
      1. Anterior and posterior convex growth arrest if younger than 5 years.
      2. Osteotomy or excision.
      3. Careful instrumentation of flexible segment of curve is an option.

3.5 Scheuermann Kyphosis

Developmental sagittal wedging of three or more adjacent vertebrae over 5 degrees. Incidence is approximately 5% of general population.

3.5.1 Clinical Features

1. Thoracic or thoracolumbar kyphosis.
2. Pain within curve, usually during growth spurt.
3. Mild scoliosis may coexist.
4. Tight hamstrings.

3.5.2 Imaging

1. Wedging of three or more vertebrae.
2. Irregularity of end plate.
3. Disk space narrowing.
4. Schmorl nodes.

3.5.3 Treatment

1. Exercise program: Strengthen abdominal and hip extensor muscles and stretch hamstrings.
2. Nonsteroidal anti-inflammatory drugs.
3. Bracing of curve if 50 to 70 degrees and skeletal maturity less than Risser 3.
4. Operative correction: Optional for curves greater than 75 degrees if pain persists or deformity is objectionable to patient.
   a) Posterior column shortening and fusion alone if flexible.
   b) Anterior release and posterior fusion if rigid.

Bibliography

1. Lonner B, Yoo A, Terran JS, et al. Effect of spinal deformity on adolescent quality of life: comparison of operative Scheuermann kyphosis, adolescent idiopathic scoliosis, and normal controls. Spine 2013;38(12):1049–1055
2. Tsirikos AI, Jain AK. Scheuermann's kyphosis; current controversies. J Bone Joint Surg Br 2011;93(7):857–864

3.6 Spondylolysis and Spondylolisthesis

Spondylolysis is the most common identifiable cause of back pain in children. The prevalence begins to plateau at around 6% by age 6 years. Etiology is a stress fracture in a susceptible pars interarticularis. The fifth lumbar vertebra is the most commonly involved. Twenty percent of pars defects are unilateral.

3.6.1 Classification

1. Dysplastic.
2. Isthmic (most common).
3. Degenerative.
4. Traumatic.
5. Pathologic.

3.6.2 Risk Factors

1. Risk factors for isthmic spondylolysis.
   a) Positive family history.
   b) Spina bifida occulta of L5.
   c) Excessive stress:
      1. Scheuermann kyphosis.
      2. Gymnastics.
      3. Athetosis.
      4. Football lineman.
2. Risk factors for progressive slip:
   a) Preadolescent age.
   b) Female.
   c) Dysplastic slip.
   d) High-grade slip (III or IV).
   e) High slip angle.

3.6.3 Signs and Symptoms

Signs and symptoms that most commonly develop in adolescence include the following.
1. Symptoms:
   a) Low back pain: Activity related; worse with extension.
   b) Pain in buttocks or proximal thighs.
2. Signs:
   a) Stiff-legged gait.
   b) Limited forward flexion.
   c) Prominent ilia.
   d) Palpable step-off of spinous process if greater than 25%.
   e) Weakness of ankle or bladder dysfunction (rare).

3.6.4 Imaging

Plain Radiographic Findings

1. Pars defect on lateral film.
2. Pars defect on oblique film (Scotty dog's neck). Does not increase diagnostic yield.
3. Elongation of pars.
4. Vertebral body slippage; measurement technique is shown in ► Fig. 3.8.
5. Relative lumbosacral kyphosis (► Fig. 3.9).

Additional Radiographic Studies

1. MRI if negative on plain films or neurologic findings present.
2. CT to visualize or confirm subtle spondylolysis.

3.6.5 Treatment

1. Activity restriction as indicated.
2. Consider brace treatment for healing of acute slip.
3. Strengthen abdominal and extensor muscles.
4. Fusion if severe pain or symptoms persist after prolonged conservative treatment, or if slip is greater than 50%.
5. Repair of defect if slip is less than 5 mm and symptomatic and patient is younger than 25 years.

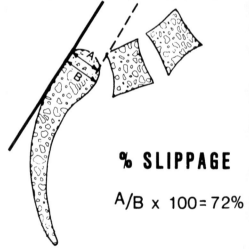

% SLIPPAGE

A/B x 100 = 72%

Fig. 3.8 Measurement of percent slip is performed with respect to a line drawn from the posterior cortex of the sacrum. Note that the reference line from the superior vertebra is parallel to the sacral line, not the L5 cortex. (Used with permission from Bradford DS. Spondylolysis and spondylolisthesis. In: Lonstein JE, Bradford DS, Winter RB, Ogilvie JW, eds. Moe's Textbook of Scoliosis and Other Spinal Deformities. 3rd ed. Philadelphia, PA: W.B. Saunders; 1995;406 (Fig. 19–5A).)

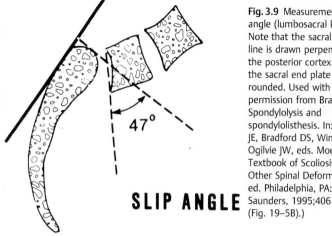

SLIP ANGLE

47°

Fig. 3.9 Measurement of slip angle (lumbosacral kyphosis). Note that the sacral reference line is drawn perpendicular to the posterior cortex because the sacral end plate may be rounded. Used with permission from Bradford DS. Spondylolysis and spondylolisthesis. In: Lonstein JE, Bradford DS, Winter RB, Ogilvie JW, eds. Moe's Textbook of Scoliosis and Other Spinal Deformities. 3rd ed. Philadelphia, PA: W.B. Saunders, 1995;406 (Fig. 19–5B).)

6. Reduction is controversial and usually considered only if slip is high grade and deformity is the primary complaint.
7. Skeletally immature patients should be followed up during growth to watch for progression.

Bibliography

1. Hu SS, Tribus CB, Diab M, Ghanayem AJ. Spondylolisthesis and spondylolysis. Instr Course Lect 2008;57:431–445

4 Miscellaneous Disorders of Growth and Development

Paul D. Sponseller

4.1 Osteochondroses

Osteochondrosis is disordered behavior of growing cartilage under load. This may include compressive or tensile loads. Most common age to present is 7 to 12 years.

4.1.1 Classification

1. Spine: Scheuermann kyphosis.
2. Upper extremity:
   a) Panner disease (capitellum).
   b) Madelung deformity (distal radial physis).
3. Lower extremity:
   a) Perthes disease.
   b) Osgood–Schlatter disease (tibial tubercle).
   c) Blount disease (medial tibial physis).
   d) Kohler disease (tarsal navicular).
   e) Freiberg disease (second metatarsal head).
   f) Sever disease (calcaneal apophysis).

4.1.2 Treatment

1. Cartilage heals and remodels with time.
2. Minimize load.
3. Bracing may help (Blount, Scheuermann).
4. Reconstruct if deformity develops (Perthes, Scheuermann, Blount, Madelung).

Bibliography

1. Crawford H. Localized disorders of bone. In: Flynn J, Weinstein SL, eds. Lovell and Winter's Pediatric Orthopaedics. 7th ed. Philadelphia, PA: Lippincott Williams & Wilkins; 2014:278–319
2. Maier GS, Lazovic D, Maus U, Roth KE, Horas K, Seeger JB. Vitamin D deficiency: the missing etiological factor in the development of juvenile osteochondrosis dissecans? J Pediatr Orthop. 2019 Jan;39(1):51-54

4.2 Musculoskeletal Tumors

Most pediatric skeletal tumors are benign. The most common primary malignancies include osteosarcoma, Ewing sarcoma, and rhabdomyosarcoma. Secondary pediatric skeletal involvement may occur with leukemia and neuroblastoma and peripheral neuroectodermal tumor.

4.2.1 Symptoms

Symptoms indicating possible malignancy include night pain that is not activity related, rapid increase in pain, increasing fatigue, or bruising.

4.2.2 Laboratory Studies

1. Erythrocyte sedimentation rate: mildly elevated for most malignant tumors.
2. Complete blood cell count: abnormal in leukemia and lymphoma.

4.2.3 Imaging

1. Plain films: Location, morphology, and host reaction are the most diagnostic features. Locations of most common benign and malignant tumors are shown in ▶ Fig. 4.1.
2. Radionuclide scans: Very sensitive for malignant bone and soft-tissue tumors; may be negative in eosinophilic granuloma.
3. CT: Best when bony changes need to be better defined.
4. MRI: Does not show bony detail well but does show soft tissue and intramedullary detail well.

4.2.4 Tumor Types

1. Benign.
   a) Eosinophilic granuloma: Reticuloendothelial lesion usually centrally located in one or several bones; poorly or well circumscribed. Usually waxes and wanes spontaneously.
   b) Osteoid osteoma: Painful nidus surrounded by sclerosis; usually found in patients aged 6 to 25 years.
   c) Osteochondroma (osteocartilaginous exostosis), metaphyseal, solitary, or multiple; growth ceases at maturity.
   d) Chondromyxoid fibroma: Eccentric local lesion, usually in lower extremity progressively enlarging. Patients aged 10 to 25 years.
   e) Chondroblastoma epiphyseal tumor of adolescence; lucent with foci of internal calcification.

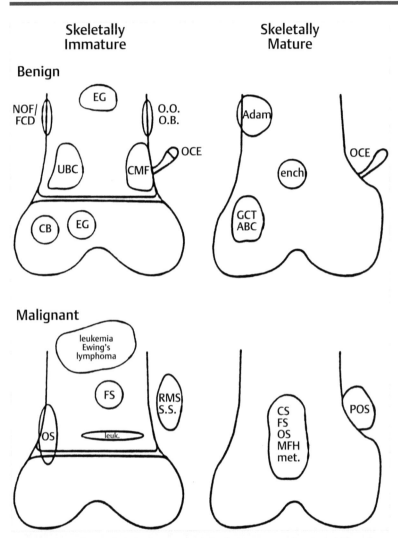

Fig. 4.1 Sites of musculoskeletal tumors in skeletally immature and mature children. See tables below for explanation of abbreviations.

   f) Unicameral bone cyst: Central lucent metaphyseal lesion usually of proximal humerus or femur; expands and thins cortex; resolves at maturity.

   g) Nonossifying fibroma: Eccentric intracortical deficit in metaphysis; resolves by maturity.

   h) Adamantinoma (Adam): Sclerotic anterior cortical deficit, usually of tibia.

   i) Enchondroma (ench) central lucent defect with internal calcification.

   j) Giant cell tumor: Lucent epimetaphyseal tumor just after maturity.

   k) Aneurysmal bone cyst: Expansile metaphyseal lesion of late adolescence that destroys cortex but leaves thin shell.

2. Malignant:

   a) Fibrosarcoma.

   b) Osteosarcoma: Most common primarily malignant bone tumor, metaphyseal; located in fastest growing regions.

   c) Chondrosarcoma: Central or peripheral, expansile tumor of young adults.

   d) Ewing sarcoma: Small cell tumor of diaphysis; patients aged 5 to 15 years; usually lasts with extensive periosteal reaction.

4.2.5 Tumors Common to Specific Locations in Children

1. Long bones (▶ Fig. 4.1).
2. Spine:
   a) Posterior elements:
      1. Aneurysmal bone cyst.
      2. Osteoid osteoma.
      3. Osteoblastoma.
   b) Vertebral body:
      1. Histiocytosis.
      2. Hemangioma.
      3. Osteosarcoma.
      4. Ewing sarcoma.
      5. Chordoma.
3. Ribs:
   a) Fibrous dysplasia.
   b) Ewing sarcoma.
   c) Chondrosarcoma.
   d) Metastasis.
4. Pelvis:
   a) Ewing sarcoma.
   b) Fibrous dysplasia.
   c) Aneurysmal bone cyst.

Table 4.1 Staging of malignant tumors

Surgical stage	Surgical grade (G)	Site (T)	Metastases (M)
IA	Low (G_1)	Intracompartmental (T_1)	M_0B
	Low (G_1)	Extracompartmental (T_2)	M_0
IIA	High (G_2)	Intracompartmental (T_1)	M_0
	High (G_2)	Extracompartmental (T_2)	M_0
III	Any	Any T	

Source: Data from Enneking WJ. Musculoskeletal Tumor Surgery. New York, NY: Churchill Livingstone; 1983.

    d) Osteoblastoma.
    e) Eosinophilic granuloma.
    f) Leukemia.
    g) Osteosarcoma.
5. Scapula:
    a) Ewing sarcoma.
    b) Osteoblastoma.
    c) Aneurysmal bone cyst.

4.2.6 Staging

1. Malignant tumors (▶ Table 4.1).
2. Benign tumors:
    a) Latent.
    b) Active.
    c) Aggressive; may expand into soft tissues or metastasize (▶ Table 4.2).

4.3 Musculoskeletal Problems in Hemophilia

Hemophilia A (factor VIII) and B (factor IX deficiency) are the two most common bleeding disorders, followed by von Willebrand disease. Factor level below 5% of normal level indicates risk of serious bleeding. These conditions should be jointly managed by hematology and orthopaedic specialists (▶ Table 4.3).

4.3.1 Treatment of Acute Hemarthropathy

1. Factor replacement, 50% every 48 hours × 6 days.
2. Aspiration.
3. Immobilization.
4. Rehabilitation.

Table 4.2 Common bone tumors

Type of tumor	Abbreviation	Name
Benign		
	EG	Eosinophilic granuloma
	OO/OB	Osteoid osteoma/osteoblastoma
	OC	Osteochondroma
	CMF	Chondromyxofibroma
	CB	Chondroblastoma
	UBC	Unicameral bone cyst
	NOF/FCD	Nonossifying fibroma/fibrous cortical defect
	Adam	Adamantinoma
	Ench	Enchondroma
	GCT	Giant cell tumor
	ABC	Aneurysmal bone cyst
Malignant		
	FS	Fibrosarcoma
	OS	Osteosarcoma
	CS	Chondrosarcoma
	MFH	Malignant fibrous histiocytoma
	POS	Parosteal osteosarcoma
	Met	Metastasis
	SS	Synovial sarcoma
	RMS	Rhabdomyosarcoma

Table 4.3 Factor doses and kinetics

Factor	Rise after one unit/kg dose (%)	Approximate half-life (h)
VIII	2	12
IX	1	24

4.3.2 Treatment of Subacute Hemarthropathy

1. Factor replacement, 30% × 2 to 6 weeks.
2. Strengthen and increase range of motion.
3. Consider synovectomy if not resolved.

4.3.3 Control of Bleeding after Fracture

1. Factor replacement, 50% × 1 to 2 days.
2. Factor replacement, 30% × 1 week.

4.3.4 Imaging (Arnold Classification)

1. Soft-tissue swelling.
2. Osteopenia, epiphyseal overgrowth.
3. Subchondral cysts; wide or square contours.
4. Irregular joint space.
5. Absent joint space.

Bibliography

1. Heyworth BE, Su EP, Figgie MP, Acharya SS, Sculco TP. Orthopedic management of hemophilia. Am J Orthop 2005;34(10):479–486
2. Zulfikar B, Koc B, Ak G, et al. Surgery in patients with von Willebrand disease. Blood Coagul Fibrinolysis 2016;27(7):812–816

4.4 Musculoskeletal Infections

4.4.1 Evaluation and Workup

Best practices:
1. Obtain all necessary cultures before starting antibiotics.
2. Blood cultures at initial workup.
3. Spinal tap if indicated in infants.
4. Aspiration of bone, joint, or abscess.
5. MRI within 24 hours if multiple tissues involved.
6. MRI scout or bone scan if it is difficult to find on physical examination.
7. Surgical drainage, if needed, under same anesthetic as MRI.
8. Multidisciplinary discussion with infectious disease and pediatrics upon admission to clarify plan.
9. Consider venous thromboembolism in children with unexpected limb swelling in setting of infection.

4.4.2 Differential Diagnosis of Infection

1. Transient synovitis.
2. Postinfectious arthritis.
3. Juvenile rheumatoid arthritis.
4. Ewing sarcoma.
5. Rheumatic fever.

4.4.3 Treatment

Empiric antibiotic recommendations by age are shown in ▶ Table 4.4.

4.4.4 Organisms

Varies with age; staphylococcal most common at all ages (▶ Table 4.5; ▶ Table 4.6).

Table 4.4 Empiric antibiotic selection for skeletal infection

Age (mo)	Antibiotic
< 1	Ampicillin/sulbactam + vancomycin
1–4	Vancomycin + ceftriaxone
> 4	Clindamycin; or vancomycin + rifampin for severe infections

Table 4.5 Organisms causing osteomyelitis

Organism	%
Staphylococcus aureus, MS	22
S. aureus, MR	22
Staphylococcus epidermidis	5
Grade A β-hemolytic streptococcus	4
Pseudomonas aeruginosa	4
Enterobacter cloacae	1
Kingella kingae	1
Streptococcus pneumoniae, Escherichia coli, enterococcus, *Candida* spp.	each < 1
No growth/unknown	38

Table 4.6 Organisms causing septic arthritis

Organism	%
Staphylococcus aureus, MS	14
S. aureus, MR	5
Group A β-hemolytic streptococcus	6
Streptococci	4
Staphylococcus epidermidis	3
Neisseria gonorrhea	2
Candida spp.	2
Haemophilus influenza	1
Group B streptococcus	1
Escherichia coli	1
Enterobacter cloacae	1
No growth/unknown	48

Bibliography

1. Copley LA. Pediatric musculoskeletal infection: trends and antibiotic recommendations. J Am Acad Orthop Surg 2009;17(10):618–626
2. Funk SS, Copley LA. Acute hematogenous osteomyelitis in children: pathogenesis, diagnosis, and treatment. Orthop Clin North Am 2017;48(2):199–208
3. Mueller AJ, Kwon JK, Steiner JW, et al. Improved magnetic resonance imaging utilization for children with musculoskeletal infection. J Bone Joint Surg Am 2015;97(22):1869–1876
4. Rosenfeld SB, Copley LA, Mignemi M, An T, Benvenuti M, Schoenecker J. Key concepts of musculoskeletal infection. Instr Course Lect 2017;66:569–584

4.5 Lyme Disease in Pediatric Orthopaedics

4.5.1 Background

1. Definition: An immune-mediated disorder in reaction to infection by the spirochete *Borrelia burgdorferi.* This disease was first characterized after an epidemic in Old Lyme, Connecticut, in the mid-1970s. Since then, other endemic areas have been identified. It may include rash, arthritis, synovitis, carditis, or neurologic manifestations.
2. It may have acute and chronic stages. Acute stage consists of rash and early arthritis. The chronic stage involves arthritis, carditis, and neuritis.
3. There are three major endemic areas in the United States:
   a) Upper mid-Atlantic area, from Maryland to Massachusetts.
   b) Upper Midwest (especially Wisconsin and Minnesota).
   c) Western states of Oregon, Utah, Nevada, and California.
4. The human leukocyte antigen (HLA)-DR4 haplotype predicts increased risk of disease.

4.5.2 Signs and Symptoms

1. Acute: Spreading rash known as erythema chronicum migrans, beginning 3 to 30 days after a tick bite.
2. Fever.
3. Headache.
4. Malaise.
5. Migratory arthralgias and myalgias.
6. Chronic swelling of large joints, most commonly the knee.

7. Involvement of one or more joints.
8. Pain, which may be minimal, as in juvenile rheumatoid arthritis, or acute, resembling bacterial arthritis.
9. Cardiac involvement, possibly including atrioventricular block or myocarditis.
10. Neurologic involvement, possibly including seventh cranial nerve (facial) palsy, meningoencephalitis, or peripheral neuropathy.

4.5.3 Physical Findings

1. Erythema chronicum migrans: spreading, oval rash.
2. Examine for cranial nerve or peripheral nerve palsy.
3. Examine all joints for effusion, even if painless.
4. Auscultate patient's heart.

4.5.4 Laboratory Tests

1. Erythrocyte sedimentation rate is usually elevated.
2. Tests for Lyme disease include two methods of antibody detection:
   a) Enzyme-linked immunosorbent assay for spirochete is sensitive but not specific. A titer of more than 1:80 is considered positive. If positive, this test should be followed by Western blot test, a gel electrophoresis technique, which is more specific.
   b) Arthrocentesis is not a specific test for Lyme disease, but it is often performed to rule out other disorders. The white blood cell count is 25,000 to 90,000 and may include up to 95% polymorphonuclear leukocytes. The spirochete is not recoverable from joint fluid.
3. Electrocardiography may be indicated to demonstrate atrioventricular block.

4.5.5 Imaging

1. Plain radiographs of the affected area are indicated.
2. Joint changes may include soft-tissue swelling in early stages, osteopenia if the inflammation has been present for several weeks, and joint space narrowing if it has been chronic.

4.5.6 Differential Diagnosis

1. Juvenile rheumatoid arthritis.
2. Bacterial arthritis.
3. Rheumatic fever.

4.5.7 Treatment

1. Consult other specialists, such as those in infectious disease, neurology, rheumatology, or cardiology, as appropriate.
2. Start treatment with oral (early stages of disease) penicillin or amoxicillin empirically.
3. Tetracycline is also an option for children who are older than 8 years. It should not be used in younger children because of potential discoloration of teeth.

4.5.8 Prognosis

Prognosis is usually good unless late joint changes or neurologic complications have occurred.

Bibliography

1. Cristofaro RL, Appel MH, Gelb RI, Williams CL. Musculoskeletal manifestations of Lyme disease in children. J Pediatr Orthop 1987;7(5):527–530
2. Milewski MD, Cruz AI Jr, Miller CP, Peterson AT, Smith BG. Lyme arthritis in children presenting with joint effusions. J Bone Joint Surg Am 2011;93(3):252–260
3. Rose CD, Fawcett PT, Eppes SC, Klein JD, Gibney K, Doughty RA. Pediatric Lyme arthritis: clinical spectrum and outcome. J Pediatr Orthop 1994;14 (2):238–241

4.6 Congenital Constriction Band Syndrome

4.6.1 Background

1. Synonyms: Amniotic band syndrome or Streeter dysplasia. The details of etiology are unknown but relate to in utero bands or strands of tissue that encircle and damage the fetus. There are four basic features of the syndrome (some or all of these may be present):
   a) Bands encircling the skin of extremities.
   b) In utero amputation of digits or portions of extremity.
   c) Acrosyndactyly (terminal syndactyly with slit-like separations proximally).
   d) Secondary effects of constriction: Nerve palsy, vascular or lymphatic occlusion, clubfoot, or other contractures.

2. Incidence: Around 1 per 5,000 live births. Upper extremities are more commonly involved than lower extremities. The incidence of clubfoot is as high as 30%. If clubfoot occurs, it may be more resistant to treatment.

4.6.2 Physical Features and Examination

All extremities should be carefully examined, especially the tips of the digits, which may have only subtle involvement. Rarely there is significant neurovascular impairment distally. In some cases, this may become worse after birth and may require urgent release of the bands. Syndactyly and hypoplastic nails are often present. The clubfoot may be paralytic if ipsilateral to a band, or it may resemble idiopathic clubfoot when contralateral.

4.6.3 Differential Diagnosis

1. Hair thread constriction may occur in infants, and the threads may be difficult to see after swelling occurs.
2. "Michelin tire baby syndrome," which is extensive and symmetrical rolls of skin.

4.6.4 Treatment

1. The constriction bands may need urgent release if there is circulatory constriction in a newborn, but this is rare.
2. Usually the bands can be excised and reconstructed when the child is 6 to 12 months of age. This can be done circumferentially at one sitting. The scarred groove should be removed until the tissues have a normal depth on either side. Dissect band off of neurovascular structures and muscle so that there is no residual constriction. The remaining edges can then be reapproximated using Z-plasty techniques so that the scar does not form a recurrent constriction.
3. Many bands are shallow enough that no surgery is needed.
4. Partial amputations may not have been completed by birth. If the tissue bridge is minimal, it can be tied off. Otherwise the amputation will need to be completed in the operating room. Amputations through bone in growing children often present later with spike formation, which requires revision.
5. Clubfoot associated with constriction band syndrome should be treated initially with the Ponseti method. The recurrence rate is significant. If multiple recurrences develop, then limited open release or tendon transfer may be indicated.

Bibliography

1. Allington NJ, Kumar SJ, Guille JT. Clubfeet associated with congenital constriction bands of the ipsilateral lower extremity. J Pediatr Orthop 1995;15 (5):599–603
2. Greene WB. One-stage release of congenital circumferential constriction bands. J Bone Joint Surg Am 1993;75(5):650–655
3. Koskimies E, Syvänen J, Nietosvaara Y, Mäkitie O, Pakkasjärvi N. Congenital constriction band syndrome with limb defects. J Pediatr Orthop 2015;35 (1):100–103

5 Skeletal Syndromes and Systemic Disorders in Pediatric Orthopaedics

Paul D. Sponseller

5.1 Introduction

This chapter summarizes developmental syndromes that involve skeletal abnormalities. It focuses on focuses on key findings and principles for each syndrome. More detailed discussion of these conditions is available in the cited references if needed.

5.2 Skeletal Dysplasias

Skeletal dysplasias involve abnormalities of bone and cartilage growth and development. Usually, short stature occurs.
1. Achondroplasia:
    a) Autosomal dominant with frequent new mutations. Most common skeletal dysplasia.
    b) Genetic defect: Fibroblast growth factor receptor protein 3 (a gain-of-function mutation).
    c) Major features:
        1. Midface hypoplasia.
        2. Rhizomelic dwarfism (limb shortening greatest proximally).
        3. Genu varum (variable).
        4. A 3- to 6-month delay in motor milestones.
        5. Thoracolumbar kyphosis, often resolving with growth.
        6. Spinal stenosis is greatest in the lumbar spine, greatest distally, but may affect entire spine, including foramen magnum, and cause severe developmental delay.
    d) Height graph (▶ Fig. 5.1).
    e) Treatment: Monitor for spinal stenosis and persistent kyphosis. Correction of knee and ankle deformities at patient's discretion. Limb lengthening is an option and is usually successful but time consuming.

Bibliography

1. Khan BI, Yost MT, Badkoobehi H, Ain MC. Prevalence of scoliosis and thoracolumbar kyphosis in patients with achondroplasia. Spine Deform 2016;4 (2):145–148

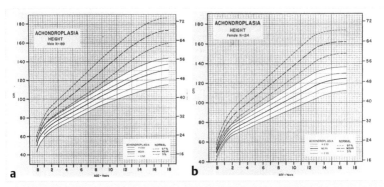

Fig. 5.1 Comparison of growth patterns of normal-stature and achondroplastic persons, in males (**a**) and females (**b**). (Used with permission from Horton WA, Rotter JI, Rimoin DL, Scott CI, Hall JG. Standard growth curves for achondroplasia. J Pediatr 1978;93 (3):436, Figs. 1 and 2.)

2. Pseudo-achondroplasia:
   a) Although these patients are also rhizomelic, the epiphyseal involvement in this syndrome causes arthrosis—a major difference from achondroplasia.
   b) Genetic defect: Cartilage oligomeric matrix protein (COMP); found in extraterritorial matrix.
   c) Major features:
      1. Rhizomelic shortening of extremities.
      2. Variable knee deformities (often varus on one side, valgus on the other).
      3. Mild platyspondyly; minimal scoliosis; no stenosis.
      4. Odontoid hypoplasia, possible C1–C2 instability.
      5. Epiphyseal deformation; eventual degeneration.
      6. Ligamentous laxity.
   d) Treatment: Screen cervical spine; correct major limb malalignment. Many patients will require joint arthroplasty as adults.
3. Diastrophic dysplasia:
   a) Autosomal recessive.
   b) Genetic defect: Diastrophic sulfate transporter (DTST).
   c) Major features:
      1. "Cauliflower ear" developing at around 6 months of age.
      2. Rhizomelic shortening of extremities.
      3. Contractures of major joints with later degenerative joint disease (DJD).
      4. Hands: Hitchhiker thumb, symphalangism.

   5. Dislocated hips: Occasionally.
   6. Equinovarus or other foot deformities.
   7. Cervical spina bifida with severe kyphosis: Sometimes resolves.
   8. Scoliosis of thoracic and lumbar spine.
   d) Treatment: Screen and monitor the cervical spine. Correct foot deformities, scoliosis, and limb contractures. Arthroplasty as indicated.
4. Spondyloepiphyseal dysplasia congenita:
   a) Autosomal dominant with frequent new mutations.
   b) Genetic defect: Collagen 2A1.
   c) Major features:
      1. *Extreme* short stature.
      2. Odontoid hypoplasia/os odontoideum: May have instability.
      3. Platyspondyly, scoliosis.
      4. Coxa vara, epiphyseal irregularity, DJD.
   d) Treatment: Screen or stabilize the cervical spine. Correct scoliosis as indicated. Treatment for hip dysplasia is of uncertain benefit. Joint arthroplasty is often indicated in adulthood.
5. Spondyloepiphyseal dysplasia tarda:
   a) Variable transmission; diagnosis late in childhood.
   b) Genetic defect: SEDL (a tracking protein) or others.
   c) Major features:
      1. Irregular ossification, DJD.
      2. Hips may resemble Perthes, but in SED bilaterally synchronous.
      3. Osteoarthritis of other joints.
      4. Scoliosis.
6. Multiple epiphyseal dysplasias:
   a) Autosomal dominant.
   b) Gene defect: COMP (found in matrix) or collagen 9 or DTST.
   c) Major features:
      1. Variable; usually mild short stature because of short limbs.
      2. Irregular epiphyseal ossification with deformity, pain, DJD.
      3. Hips, knees, and ankles are most involved. Patella may show "double layer."
      4. Usually presents in late childhood to adulthood.
7. Metatropic dysplasia:
   a) Major features:
      1. Epiphyseal or metaphyseal enlargement: "Knobby" joints with contractures.
      2. Cervical stenosis, instability.
      3. Scoliosis, kyphosis, later onset.
      4. Coccygeal tail.
      5. Thoracic hypoplasia; may cause respiratory compromise.

      6. Initially short-limb dwarfism; becomes short-trunk type with onset of scoliosis.

8. Chondrodysplasia punctata (Conradi–Hünermann syndrome).
   a) Autosomal dominant, recessive, and X-linked.
   b) Major features:
      1. Multiple asymmetric epiphyseal calcifications.
      2. Rhizomelic form may have cervical stenosis or kyphosis as well as thoracolumbar scoliosis.
      3. Good prognosis for dominant form. Decreased life expectancy for other forms.

9. Multiple hereditary exostoses (MHE):
   a) Inheritance: Autosomal dominant.
   b) Genetic defect: At least three have been described; EXT-1 and -2 on different chromosomes. EXT-1 produces more serious form.
   c) Clinical appearance: Mild short stature.
   d) Categories of problems:
      1. Local impingement on tendons, nerves, spinal canal, and ribs.
      2. Asymmetrical growth in two-bone segments (forearms and legs) leading to valgus at knees, ankles, elbow, and wrists and possibly radial head dislocation.
      3. Leg-length inequality (usually < 4 cm).
      4. Risk of malignant degeneration (in about 1% of patients).
      5. Osteochondromas may grow silently in spinal canal; monitor neurologic examination.
      6. Patients with MHE often heal incisions with wide scars or keloids.
   e) Radiographic features:
      1. Osteochondromas in metaphysis, pointing away from joint.
      2. Cortex of osteochondroma is confluent with that of host bone.
      3. May be sessile or pedunculated.
   f) Treatment:
      1. Resect lesions only when symptomatic. Increased rotation not predictable in forearm.
      2. Correct knee and ankle valgus when greater than 10 degrees.
      3. Monitor in adulthood every 2 years, possibly with bone scan.
      4. Obtain spine MRI when patient is old enough to undergo without anesthesia, or if there is any question of involvement.

10. Dysplasia epiphysialis hemimelica (Trevor disease):
    a) Definition: Epiphyseal osteochondroma; no genetic pattern.
    b) Clinical features: Presents in the first decade of life; restricted joint motion, enlarged joint, or locking. Knee, foot, and ankle are most commonly involved.

c) Radiographs: Multiple opacities in exostotic cartilage; these eventually coalesce.

d) Treatment: Resection, attempting to preserve normal cartilage.

Bibliography

1. Kettelkamp DB, Campbell CJ, Bonfiglio M. Dysplasia epiphysealis hemimelica. A report of fifteen cases and a review of the literature. J Bone Joint Surg Am 1966;48(4):746–765, discussion 765–766

11. Multiple enchondromas (Ollier disease):
    a) Genetic defect: *PTH/PTHRP*.
    b) Clinical presentation:
        1. Angular deformity.
        2. Bony irregularity.
        3. Limb-length inequality.
    c) Radiographic features:
        1. Diffuse enchondromas in metaphysis; occasionally epiphyses. Usually asymmetrical.
    d) Treatment:
        a) Angular or length correction of limb.
        b) Monitor for malignancy, especially in Maffucci syndrome.
12. Cleidocranial dysplasia:
    a) Autosomal dominant.
    b) Genetic defect: *CBFA1*, a transcription factor.
    c) Clinical features:
        1. Persistently open skull sutures with bulging calvarium.
        2. Hypoplasia or aplasia of clavicles.
        3. Wide symphysis pubis.
        4. Hip abnormalities (coxa vara).
        5. Short middle phalanx of fifth finger.
        6. Scoliosis with or without syringomyelia.
        7. Multiple dental abnormalities.

Bibliography

1. Brigham EM, Hennrikus WL. Like father, like son: cleidocranial dysplasia: a case report. JBJS Case Connect 2015;5(4):e94
2. Jensen BL. Somatic development in cleidocranial dysplasia. Am J Med Genet 1990;35(1):69–74

13. Dyschondrosteosis (Léri–Weill disorder):
   a) Genetic defect: *SHOX* pseudoautosomal genes.
   b) Major features:
      1. Mild short stature (< 25 percentile).
      2. Madelung deformity (dorsoulnar deficiency of distal radial growth).
      3. Relative shortening of forearm and leg; varus or valgus deformity.
      4. Females predominant.

5.3 Other Syndromes Involving Short Stature

5.3.1 Cornelia de Lange (Brachmann de Lange Type)

1. Genetic defect: *NIPBL* or microdeletion on chromosome 3.
2. Major features:
   a) Synophrys (single eyebrow).
   b) Down-turned mouth.
   c) Mandibular spur in infancy.
   d) Hirsutism.
   e) Gastroesophageal reflux.
   f) Small for gestational age, with continued growth retardation.
   g) Motor, speech, and intellectual delay.
   h) Cardiac abnormalities.
3. Orthopaedic involvement:
   a) Upper extremity anomalies (~100%):
      1. Micromelia, phocomelia.
      2. Decreased number of fingers.
      3. Lobster-claw hand.
      4. Proximally placed thumb.
      5. Elbow anomalies.
   b) Lower extremities:
      1. Miscellaneous foot deformities and contracture.
      2. Avascular necrosis (AVN) of femoral head in 10%.
4. Treatment: Correct lower extremity abnormalities if limiting ambulation; upper extremities: individualized treatment.

5.3.2 Riley–Day Familial Dysautonomia

1. Ashkenazi Jews only: Autosomal recessive.
2. Sympathetic overactivity is key feature.
3. Major features:
   a) Deficient sensation of pain and proprioception.
   b) Gastroesophageal reflux, pneumonia.
   c) Variable life expectancy.

4. Orthopaedic abnormalities and implications:
    a) Scoliosis/kyphosis before age 8; poor brace tolerance; fuse early.
    b) Fractures from osteopenia or dyscoordination.
    c) AVN of femoral head, distal femur, talus.
    d) Hip dysplasia.

5.3.3 Nail–Patella Syndrome

1. Autosomal dominant, normal life expectancy.
2. Orthopaedic features:
    a) Nails grooved, small, or absent, especially on thumb.
    b) Multiple knee anomalies: Patella tripartite, small, or absent, lateral femoral condyle hypoplastic, (valgus) osteochondritis dissecans of lateral femur and talus.
    c) Elbow: Capitellar hypoplasia, cubitus valgus, flexion contracture.
    d) Iliac horns.
    e) X-linked hypophosphatemic rickets.

5.4 Sclerosing Bone Disorders

1. Fibrodysplasia ossificans progressiva
    a) Progressive, disabling heterotopic ossification or ankylosis. Incidence—1:1,000,000.
    b) Etiology: Enhanced signaling of *BMP4*.
    c) Characteristic shortening/valgus of great toe (▶ Fig. 5.2).
    d) Ossification starts as tender, hard nodule; progresses proximal to distal, posterior to anterior.
    e) Do not biopsy; may accelerate the process.
    f) Genetics: Usually a spontaneous mutation but may be transmitted as autosomal dominant.
2. Progressive diaphyseal dysplasia (Camurati–Engelmann disease):
    a) Clinical features: Pain, fatigue, muscle atrophy
    b) Etiology: Activating mutation in transforming growth factor beta (TGF-β) genes.
    c) Radiographs: Symmetrically widened, sclerotic diaphyses and epiphyses, spared tibia, femur most commonly involved.
    d) Treatment: Osteotomies only if marked deformity. Possible role for bisphosphonates.
3. Melorheostosis:
    a) Syndrome involving asymmetrical extraosseous longitudinal hyperostotic streaks resembling molten wax; limb pain and soft-tissue contracture.
    b) Treatment: Analgesics, bracing contracture releases, and bone shortening.

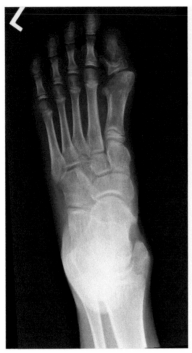

Fig. 5.2 Characteristic shortening/alus of great toe in Fibrodysplasia Ossificans Progressiva.

4. Osteopathia striata:
   a) Linear intraosseous metaphyseal striations.
   b) Autosomal dominant.
   c) Asymptomatic.
   d) No treatment required.
5. Osteopoikilosis:
   a) Multiple symmetrical intraosseous epiphyseal–metaphyseal "spots."
   b) Autosomal dominant.
   c) Asymptomatic.

5.5 Fibrous Dysplasia

1. Background: Inheritance—somatic mutation that produces mosaic distribution of lesions in one (monostotic) or many (polyostotic) bones:
   a) The molecular basis is a postzygotic activating mutation in the *GNAS1* gene, which encodes for the cyclic adenosine monophosphatase–regulating α subunit of the Gs protein complex.

  b) Histologically, the fibrous tissue undergoes ossification to small, irregular trabeculae ("alphabet soup"). The disease process is most active during growth and causes weakening of the bone and pathologic fracture.
2. Clinical manifestations: Monostotic form accounts for 80% of cases. Polyostotic is found in several bones on one side of the skeleton or scattered throughout the skeleton. In the axial skeleton, the craniofacial bones and the ribs are the most common sites; in the appendicular skeleton, the tibia and proximal femur are the most common sites.
  a) Monostotic fibrous dysplasia usually presents without symptoms, and the lesion is found when a radiograph is taken for unrelated reasons.
  b) Polyostotic fibrous dysplasia often results in distortion of the skeletal and facial configuration. The peak incidence of fractures is during the first decade of life, followed by a decrease thereafter. Lesions of the femoral neck may cause progressive coxa vara, leading to the shepherd's crook deformity; this is the most common angular deformity in polyostotic fibrous dysplasia. Spinal involvement and scoliosis may also occur.
  c) Skin lesions include café-au-lait spots with an irregular border ("coast of Maine").
  d) Fibrous dysplasia may be associated with significant endocrine disturbances: hyperthyroidism, phosphaturia, precocious puberty, and diabetes mellitus. The McCune–Albright syndrome includes the triad of polyostotic fibrous dysplasia, café-au-lait spots, and precocious puberty.
3. Imaging findings: Elongated lesion with symmetric cortical thinning and outward expansion, the characteristic of diaphyseal "long lesion in a long bone." Lesion shows few trabecular markings and has a ground-glass appearance. Some may be entirely radiolytic or radiodense. There may be an associated angular deformity. Fibrous dysplasia shows excessive uptake on bone scan.
4. Treatment: Unnecessary for asymptomatic lesions of fibrous dysplasia. Large or symptomatic lesions may be treated by curettage and allografting. Lesions of the femoral neck should be treated with metallic support with or without cortical bone grafting because of the risk of fatigue fracture. If symptomatic varus deformity is present, then treatment should include valgus osteotomy with cortical bone grafting and rigid internal fixation. Because of poor bone quality, intramedullary fixation is preferable to plates and screws alone for lesions of the femoral shaft. Deformity may occur at stress risers, similar to osteogenesis imperfecta. Medical management includes the use of bisphosphonates. Early studies suggest that bisphosphonates decrease pain, improve the radiologic appearance of the lesions, and decrease the fracture rate.

5.6 Marfan and Related Disorders

5.6.1 Marfan Syndrome (MFS)

1. This is a disorder of fibrillin-1, which also affects TGF-β distribution and has multiple effects on the skeleton and connective tissue. Because some features may be seen in the general population, the following diagnostic criteria have been developed.
2. Diagnostic (Ghent) criteria: Two major criteria and involvement of another system. The asterisks below indicate major manifestations, of which there are four possibilities.
   a) Genetic: MFS diagnosis in first-degree relative or fibrillin gene mutation known to cause MFS.*
   b) Skeletal:
      1. Pectus excavatum or carinatum.
      2. Dolichostenomelia (long, narrow limbs; arm span–height > 1.05).
      3. Arachnodactyly (long, narrow digits with positive thumb and wrist sign). "Thumb" or Steinberg sign is when the entire distal phalanx of the thumb protrudes beyond the ulnar border of the clenched fist. "Wrist" or Walker–Murdoch sign is positive when the thumb can overlap the nail of the fifth finger when clasping the opposite wrist (▶ Fig. 5.3).
      4. Vertebral column deformity (increased kyphosis, scoliosis > 20 degrees).
      5. Significant hindfoot valgus.
      6. Facial features including a high narrow cranium, down-slanting eyes, narrowly arched palate.
      7. Elbow flexion contracture.
      8. Protrusio acetabula.
   c) Ocular (*major involvement if any four of the skeletal features below are present):
      1. *Ectopia lentis (superolateral dislocation).
      2. Flat cornea.
      3. Retinal detachment.
      4. Myopia.
   d) Cardiovascular:
      1. *Dilation of aortic root with ascending arch aneurysm.
      2. *Aortic dissection: Usually ascending segment.
      3. Aortic valve regurgitation.
      4. Mitral valve regurgitation.
      5. Abdominal aortic aneurysm.
   e) Pulmonary:
      1. Spontaneous pneumothorax.
      2. Apical bleb.

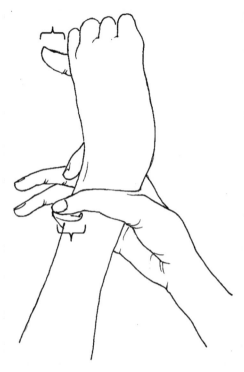

Fig. 5.3 Illustration of the thumb and wrist signs. Thumb sign: The entire distal phalanx of the thumb protrudes beyond the ulnar border of the clenched fist. Wrist sign: Thumb covers the entire fifth fingernail when wrapped around the opposite wrist.

   f) Skin:
      1. Striae atrophicae ("stretch marks").
      2. Hernia.
   g) Central nervous system:
      1. Dural ectasia.
      2. Learning disability.
      3. Hyperactivity.
3. Implications:
   a) Monitor aortic and cardiac status.
   b) β-Blocker or losartan for aortic dilation.
   c) Restrict from vigorous exertion.
   d) Counsel regarding genetics.
   e) Treat skeletal deformity if symptomatic. Bracing does not usually control spinal deformity.

5.6.2 Homocystinuria

This disorder may be mistaken for MFS but is most readily distinguished by mental retardation. It has the following major features:

1. Mental retardation.
2. Dislocated lens (inferomedial).
3. Arachnodactyly.
4. Joint stiffness.
5. Cavus feet.
6. Scoliosis or kyphosis.
7. Diagnosis: Urine amino acid screen.
8. Treatment: Vitamin B6 administration, methionine restriction.

5.6.3 Congenital Contractural Arachnodactyly (Beals Syndrome)

1. This is also an MFS look alike, so much so that the original MFS patient had this syndrome.
2. Genetic defect: Fibrillin-2.
3. Clinical features:
   a) Face: Oval with recessed jaw, flattened ears.
   b) Eyes: Occasional intraocular coloboma.
   c) Heart: Congenital septal and valve defects.
   d) Skeleton: Flexion contractures, which partially improve with time.
   e) Hands: Contracture of proximal interphalangeal and distal interphalangeal joints.
   f) Scoliosis: Appears by mid-childhood.

5.6.4 Achard Syndrome

1. Clinical features:
   a) Arachnodactyly.
   b) Generalized ligamentous laxity.
   c) Mandibular hypoplasia.

5.6.5 Stickler Syndrome (Hereditary Arthro-ophthalmopathy)

1. Genetic etiology: A mutation in type II collagen.
2. Clinical features:
   a) Progressive myopia beginning in first decade.
   b) Retinal detachment.

c) Abnormal epiphyseal development, eventual DJD. May resemble Perthes.
d) With or without mild joint hypermobility.
e) With or without marfanoid habitus.
f) Autosomal dominant.

Bibliography

1. Beals RK. Hereditary arthro-ophthalmopathy (the Stickler syndrome). Report of a kindred with protrusio acetabuli. Clin Orthop Relat Res 1977;125(125):32–35

5.6.6 MASS (Mitral Valve Prolapse, Aortic Anomalies, Skin and Skeleton Changes) Phenotype

1. An overlap connective tissue disorder.
2. Genetic etiology: Unknown/variable.
3. Clinical characteristics: Mitral valve, aortic root, skin, and skeleton.

5.6.7 Shprintzen–Goldberg Syndrome

1. Clinical syndrome of connective tissue.
2. Genetic defect: Fibrillin 1.
3. Clinical features: Craniosynostosis, exophthalmos, low-set ears, arachnodactyly, camptodactyly, and developmental delay.

5.6.8 Loeys–Dietz Syndrome

1. Connective tissue disorder characterized by triad of hypertelorism, arterial tortuosity and aneurysms, and bifid uvula.
2. Genetic defect: TGF-β receptor protein 1 or 2 or related proteins.
3. Other clinical features: Clubfeet or skewfeet, knee and elbow hyperextensibility, bifid anterior or posterior arch of C1, cervical instability, scoliosis, and dural ectasia.
4. Treatment: Screen for aneurysms; rule out cervical instability; consider angiotensin-converting enzyme inhibitor. Conservative treatment preferred for feet. Spine treatment as for MFS.

5.7 Arthrogryposis/Contracture

1. Arthrogryposis multiplex congenita:
    a) This is the classic contractural syndrome seen by orthopaedists.
    b) Etiology is unknown; likely multifactorial.

c) Major features are skeletal and may affect all four limbs, just uppers, or just lowers. Involvement is usually greatest distally within each limb.
   1. Hips: Frequently dislocated. Contractures are usually into abduction and external rotation.
   2. Knees: Flexion more common than extension.
   3. Clubfoot, vertical talus: Common, often resistant to cast treatment.
   4. Upper extremities: Often extended at elbows: adducted, stiff fingers.
   5. Spine: Paralytic scoliosis, torticollis.
d) Treatment:
   1. Joint range of motion can be shifted but not increased. Stretching and splinting are indicated.
   2. Guided growth procedures early; osteotomies most useful near end of growth.
   3. Knee and hip repositioning osteotomies may improve function.
   4. Fractures common after manipulation or cast.
2. Larsen syndrome:
   a) Genetic defect: Filamin gene (*FLNB*).
   b) Orthopaedic features:
      1. Dislocated hips, hyperextended or dislocated knees.
      2. Clubfeet, vertical tali, or other foot deformities.
      3. Normal muscle mass.
      4. Elbow dislocations.
      5. Cervical kyphosis and instability; may cause paresis.
      6. Thoracic and lumbar scoliosis.
   c) Nonorthopaedic features:
      1. Flattened face; depressed, widened nasal bridge.
      2. Cleft palate.
   d) Treatment: Surgically correct and stabilize cervical kyphosis if present. Correct hips, knees, and feet using standard principles to maximize function.
3. Freeman–Sheldon (whistling face) syndrome:
   a) Genetics: Recessive or dominant; mechanisms unknown.
   b) Clinical findings:
      1. Small mouth and chin (may cause difficulty with intubation).
      2. Fingers arthrogrypotic, flexed and ulnar deviated.
      3. Clubfeet or vertical talus.
      4. Scoliosis/kyphosis.
4. Mobius syndrome:
   a) Congenital facial diplegia.
   b) Variable absence of shoulder girdle muscles.
   c) Clubfeet and hand contractures or anomalies.
5. Pterygium syndromes:
   a) Multiple pterygium (Escobar) syndrome:

1. Genetic defect: Acetylcholine receptor.
2. Static disorder with flexion contractures and webs at all flexion creases.
3. Short stature.
4. Congenital spinal anomalies.
5. Treatment: Judicious guided growth and osteotomies.
b) Popliteal pterygium syndrome:
   1. Webs only across perineum and knees.
   2. Facial malformations.
   3. Contractures are due to a single cord from ischium to calcaneus, with nerve bow-strung across the joint.

5.8 Vascular Abnormalities

5.8.1 Klippel–Trenaunay–Weber

1. Clinical features:
   a) Cutaneous hemangioma (port-wine stain).
   b) Varicose veins.
   c) Limb hypertrophy: width or length.
2. Genetic basis: None known.
3. Treatment:
   a) Initially treated with compressive therapy.
   b) Focal limb deformity treated as needed.

5.8.2 Maffucci Syndrome

1. Defect in parathyroid receptor protein.
2. Major features:
   a) Multiple enchondromata.
   b) Limb shortening and deformity.
   c) Cavernous hemangiomas.
   d) Risk of sarcomatous transformation.

5.8.3 Sturge–Weber Syndrome

1. Major features:
   a) Port-wine hemangioma in trigeminal distribution.
   b) Neurologic sequelae resulting from meningeal hemangioma.

5.8.4 Blue Rubber Bleb Nevus Syndrome

1. Autosomal dominant.

2. Clinical features:
   a) Bluish cavernous hemangiomata on trunk, upper arms.
      1. May bleed from gastrointestinal tract locations.
      2. May cause pain.
   b) Regional hyperhidrosis.

5.8.5 Kasabach–Merritt Syndrome

1. Clinical features:
   a) Solitary or multiple cavernous hemangiomas on the trunk or extremities.
   b) Consumptive coagulopathy secondary to above.

5.8.6 Ataxia–Telangiectasia (Louis–Bar)

1. Clinical features:
   a) Telangiectasia on conjunctivae, face, neck, and arms.
   b) Progressive ataxia and dysarthria.
   c) Skeletal problems: Equinovarus or valgus feet, scoliosis, limited ambulation.
   d) Immunodeficiency, infection, and cancer risk.
   e) Increased sensitivity to ionizing radiation.
   f) Decreased life expectancy.
   g) Genetics: Autosomal recessive. Defect in *AT1* gene; related to immunoglobulin superfamily.

5.8.7 Hemophilia A (see also Chapter 4)

1. Deficiency of factor VIII. X-linked inheritance. Males are affected, and females are carriers.
2. Clinical features: Bleeding into muscles, joints, and central nervous system. Often first noted at circumcision.
   a) Factor VIII level less than 1%, severe; 2 to 5%, moderate; and greater than 5%, mild.
   b) After several bleeds, joints develop synovial hypertrophy and are prone to rebleeds (target joints).
   c) Most common target joints: Knees, ankles, elbows, and shoulders.
3. Treatment: Prevent target joint by early aspiration, irrigation, and rest. Hemophilic arthropathy: Joint effusion present for over 6 weeks. Consider synovectomy. Severe arthritis, consider joint replacement.

5.8.8 Sickle Cell Anemia

1. Disorder of β chains of hemoglobin. Hemoglobin S is a point mutation replacing a glutamic acid to valine. Hemoglobin C replaces this with lysine at the same position. S mutation is present in 1:500 African Americans. Hemoglobin SS produces severe sickling.
    a) Hemoglobin SC produces moderate sickling.
    b) Sickle–thalassemia produces mild sickling.
    c) Sickle cell trait is heterozygous; one normal and one S globin inherited; no clinical sickling.
2. Clinical features:
    a) Dactylitis: Swelling of digits in infants.
    b) Sickle crisis: Infarcts of muscle, bone, other tissue.
    c) Growth, maturation diminished or delayed.
    d) Infections with *Salmonella* or *Staphylococcus* spp.
3. Treatment:
    a) Rehydration, analgesics.
    b) Transfusion.
    c) Core decompression for early AVN.

5.9 Overgrowth Syndromes

5.9.1 Generalized Bodily Overgrowth

1. Prader–Willi
    a) Partial deletion of paternal chromosome 15.
    b) Major findings:
        1. Infantile hypotonia.
        2. Obesity beginning after age 1.
        3. Mental retardation.
        4. Cryptorchidism.
        5. Short stature.
        6. Eyes slant upward and lateral.
    c) Orthopaedic findings:
        1. Developmental dysplasia of the hip: 10%.
        2. Scoliosis: 50%.
        3. Small hands and feet.
    d) Treatment: Growth hormone improves growth and muscle mass.
2. Bardet–Biedl:
    a) Multiple genetic mutations may be causative.
    b) Major findings:
        1. Truncal obesity.
        2. Mental retardation.

    3. Hypogonadism.

    4. Retinitis pigmentosa.

    5. Renal abnormalities.

  c) Orthopaedic abnormalities:

    1. Postaxial polydactyly (feet more than hands).

3. Beckwith–Wiedemann:

  a) Autosomal dominant; partial deletion of chromosome 15.

  b) Major findings:

    1. Large stature.

    2. Omphalocele.

    3. Macroglossia (may partially regress).

    4. Hypoglycemia.

    5. Multiple organ enlargement; risk of Wilms tumor. Ultrasound every 3 months until age 7.

  c) Orthopaedic abnormalities:

    1. Leg-length inequality.

    2. Neurologic damage if hypoglycemia not controlled.

    3. Polydactyly, idiopathic scoliosis, radial head dislocation variable.

5.9.2 Asymmetric Overgrowth

1. Idiopathic hemihypertrophy:

  a) Skeletal findings:

    1. One side of the body larger in all dimensions.

    2. Growth proportionate over time.

    3. Lower extremities most often affected; trunk and upper extremities may or may not be affected.

  b) Genitourinary system:

    1. Wilms tumor (nephroblastoma): Around 5%.

    2. Medullary sponge kidney.

    3. Renal malposition.

  c) Vascular system: Aortic, cerebral vascular, or congenital heart abnormalities,

2. Russell–Silver syndrome:

  a) Genetically heterogeneous.

  b) Short stature.

  c) Small, triangular face; may be asymmetrical.

  d) Genitourinary and genital malformations.

  e) Orthopaedic features:

    1. Hemihypertrophy.

    2. Other miscellaneous skeletal findings (pseudoepiphysis of second metacarpal, clinodactyly).

3. Goldenhar syndrome (hemifacial microsomia, oculoauriculovertebral dysplasia)
   a) Usually not inherited.
   b) Major features:
      1. Epibulbar dermoids.
      2. Preauricular skin tags; facial asymmetry.
   c) Orthopaedic abnormalities:
      1. Congenital vertebral anomalies.
      2. Other aspects of VATER (vertebral defects, imperforate anus, tracheoesophageal fistula, radial and renal dysplasia) association.
   d) Implications: Monitor for scoliosis; be aware of difficult intubation.
4. Klippel–Feil syndrome:
   a) Key feature:
      1. Cervical spine fusions; may have stenosis; instability.
   b) Genetics: Usually sporadic; rarely inherited.
   c) Possible skeletal associations:
      1. Congenital or "idiopathic" scoliosis of lower spine: 60% of patients.
      2. Sprengel deformity (30%).
      3. Upper extremity and hand anomalies.
   d) Nonskeletal associations:
      1. Genitourinary and renal malformations.
      2. Hearing impairment.
      3. Cardiac anomalies.
      4. Facial asymmetry.
   e) Implications:
      1. Screen early for hearing impairment, genitourinary malformations (ultrasound).
      2. Look for other skeletal malformations.
      3. Counsel regarding activity and anesthesia if neck is unstable.
5. Proteus syndrome:
   a) A hamartomatous disorder affecting all three germ layers. Most likely a postzygotic mutation.
   b) Characterized by its variability and progressive nature, named after Greek god able to change shape at will.
   c) Macrodactyly, asymmetrical tissue overgrowth, and nevi are key features.
   d) Definitive diagnosis can be established by scoring, as in ▶ Table 5.1.
   e) Treatment: Restoration of alignment by epiphysiodesis, osteotomy.

Table 5.1 Proteus syndrome

Diagnostic criteria	Points
Macrodactyly and/or hemihypertrophy	5
Thickening of skin	4
Lipomas and subcutaneous tumors	4
Verrucous epidermal nevus	3
Macrocephaly	2.5
Other minor abnormalities	1

Note: Definitive diagnosis is made if score is ≥ 13 points; questionable diagnosis, 10–13 points; diagnosis excluded, < 10 points.

5.10 Neurofibromatosis Type 1

Neurofibromatosis type 1 (NF-1) is the most prevalent skeletal disorder caused by a single gene defect. The gene, *NF1*, codes for neurofibromin. It is involved in the GTPase activating protein pathway and has tumor-suppressive function.

5.10.1 Diagnosis

At least two of the following criteria of the National Institutes of Health:
1. Café-au-lait spots (six or more spots ≥ 1.5 cm after puberty or ≥ 0.5 cm before puberty).
2. Subcutaneous NF.
3. Positive biopsy.
4. Positive family history (first-degree relative affected).
5. Skeletal manifestation:
   a) Long-bone pseudarthrosis.
   b) Dystrophic curve of spine.
   c) Elephantiasis neuromatosa.
6. Optic glioma.
7. Two or more Lisch nodules (hamartomas in iris).
8. Axillary or inguinal freckling.

5.10.2 Features of Dystrophic Spinal Curve

1. Severe apical rotation or wedging.
2. Paravertebral mass.
3. "Spindling" of transverse process.
4. Thinning of rib.
5. Foraminal enlargement.
6. Vertebral scalloping (▶ Fig. 5.4).

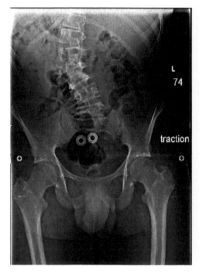

Fig. 5.4 Severe focal apical vertebral wedging, scalloping in NF1.

L
74

traction

5.10.3 Orthopaedic Implications

1. Bracing is not effective for dystrophic curves.
2. Dystrophic curves require more aggressive treatment (fuse if 50 degrees; consider anterior and posterior if > 70 degrees or kyphosis > 50 degrees).
3. Preoperative MRI or computed tomography/myelogram on all dystrophic curves.
4. Rule out sarcoma if unexplained pain or localized growth occurs.

5.11 Ehlers–Danlos Syndromes

This group of connective tissue abnormalities has at least 11 different subtypes. Beighton later suggested six descriptive types (classic, hypermobility, vascular, scoliotic, arthrochalasis, and dermatosparaxis) and five unspecified types. Many other patients do not fit precisely into one of the groups. Most are disorders of collagen types 1 and 5, or their processing enzymes. They are listed in ▶ Table 5.2.

The Beighton score is used to rate hypermobility; see ▶ Table 5.3.

Table 5.2 Types of Ehlers-Danlos syndrome

Names	Type	Genetics	Skeletal manifestations			Other problems
			Dislocations	Joint laxity	Scoliosis	
Classic: gravis	1	AD	+	+	+	Aneurysms, viscus rupture, hernias
Classic: mitis	2	AD	−	+/−	−	—
Benign hypermobile	3	AD	+	+	−	Mitral valve prolapse
Vascular	4	AD/AR	+	Fingers	−	Aneurysms, spontaneous rupture
Unspecified X-linked	5	X	−	−	−	Intramuscular hemorrhage, "floppy baby"
Ocular–scoliotic	6	AR	+	+	+ +	Ocular complications
Arthrochalasis multiplex	7	AR	+	+	+	Short stature
Unspecified: periodontosis	8	AD	−	+/−	−	Necrobiosis of skin; periodontosis
Unspecified: occipital horn	9	X	+	+	-	Occipital horns, skeletal dysplasia
Unspecified: platelet dysfunction	10	AR	−	Hands	−	Platelet defect
Unspecified: familial laxity	11	AD	Patellae, hips		+	

Abbreviations: AD, autosomal dominant; AR, autosomal recessive.

Table 5.3 Beighton score: a score ≥ 4 out of a possible 9 indicates hypermobility

Movement type	Left	Right
Finger metacarpophalangeal joint hyperextends beyond 90 degrees	1 point	1
Thumb apposes to volar surface of forearm	1	1
Elbow hyperextends beyond 10 degrees	1	1
Knee hyperextends beyond 10 degrees	1	1
Palms may be placed flat on floor with forward bend with knees straight	1	

5.12 Osteogenesis Imperfecta

Osteogenesis imperfecta comprises a group of disorders of type I collagen causing bone fragility and in some cases blue sclerae, hearing loss, and abnormal dentin. The osseous fragility tends to improve after puberty.

5.12.1 Sillence Classification Types

1. Type I:
    a) Variable osseous fragility (minimal though moderately severe).
    b) Blue sclerae (at all ages).
    c) Early hearing loss.
    d) Autosomal dominant.
2. Type II (lethal perinatal osteogenesis imperfecta): Extremely severe osseous fragility, with stillbirth or neonatal death:
    a) Subgroup A—Radiographs show broad, crumpled long bones and broad ribs with continuous beading. Autosomal dominant or new mutation.
    b) Subgroup B—Radiographs show broad crumpled long bones, ribs show discontinuous beading or are not beaded. Autosomal recessive.
    c) Subgroup C—Radiographs show thin, fractured long bones and thin, beaded ribs. Autosomal recessive.
3. Type III:
    a) Autosomal recessive.
    b) Fractures at birth, then progressive deformity.
    c) Normal sclerae and hearing.
4. Type IV:
    a) Moderate osseous fragility.
    b) Normal sclerae (blue in infancy).
    c) Variable deformity of long bones and spine.
    d) Autosomal dominant.

Note that the value of opalescent dentin for subcategorization of osteogenesis imperfecta is uncertain.

5.12.2 Additional Types (after Sillence)

1. Type V:
   a) Hyperplastic callus.
   b) Radial head dislocation.
   c) Moderate fracture rate.
   d) Normal type I collagen.
2. Type VI:
   a) Moderate osseous fragility.
   b) "Fish-scale" pattern of lamellae on histology.
   c) Excessive osteoid deposition.
   d) Normal type I collagen.
3. Type VII:
   a) Rhizomelic short stature.
   b) Normal type I collagen.
   c) CRTAP (cartilage-associated protein) defect.
   d) Reported only in Canadian First Nations Community.
4. Type VIII:
   a) Short stature and normal sclerae.
   b) Bulbous metaphyses.
   c) Extreme osteopenia.
   d) Normal type I collagen; attributable to defect in leprecan, which hydroxylates proline #986 of COL 1A1.

Treatment options are the same for all types (I through VIII):
1. Bisphosphonates if frequent fractures.
2. Telescoping rods for bowing of long bones if function is limited.
3. Encourage standing and walking when feasible.
4. Minimize use of plate fixation in growing children.
5. Spine correction if scoliosis is severe and progressive.
6. Stabilize and decompress basilar invagination if symptomatic.

5.12.3 Bruck Syndrome

1. Osteogenesis imperfecta with multiple congenital contractures.
2. Genetic defect in bone-specific telopeptide lysyl hydroxylase.
3. Contractures of knees, feet and ankles, elbows.

5.13 Mucopolysaccharidoses

Mucopolysaccharidoses are recessive disorders of glycosaminoglycan (mucopolysaccharide) storage, all autosomal recessive. They have delayed appearance of signs and symptoms corresponding to the accumulation of storage products. Most are progressive. ▶ Table 5.4 describes their features.

Table 5.4 The mucopolysaccharidoses

Number	Name	Genetics	Enzyme defect	Clinical features
I-H	Hurler	AR	μ-L-iduronidase	Diagnosis at 1–3 y; corneal clouding, MR, kyphoscoliosis. Some amelioration with enzyme replacement, BMT, gene therapy
I-S	Scheie	AR	μ-L-iduronidase	Corneal clouding, aortic abnormality, normal intelligence, longer survival
II	Hunter	XR	Iduronate sulfate sulfatase	Clear cornea, mild MR, ± kyphosis
III	Sanfilippo A, B, C, D	AR		Dementia, seizures
IV-A	Morquio-A	AR	B galactosidase —6-sulfate sulfatase (increased urinary keratan sulfate)	Short trunk, odontoid hypoplasia with cervical instability, flame-shaped vertebrae, kyphosis (TL)
IV-B	Morquio-B	AR	B galactosidase	Milder form
VI	Maroteaux–Lamy	AR	Arylsulfatase B	Corneal clouding, normal intelligence, ± cervical stenosis, ± TL kyphosis
VII	Sly	AR	B-glucuronidase	May have epiphyseal dysplasia

Abbreviations: AR, autosomal recessive; BMT, bone marrow transplant; MR, mental retardation; TL, thoracolumbar; XR, X-linked recessive.

5.14 Malformations of the Hand and Foot

5.14.1 Syndactyly

1. Terminology:
   a) Extent: Partial or complete.
   b) Simple: Skin only.
   c) Complex: Synostosis.
   d) Polysyndactyly: Hidden duplicated skeletal structures.
   e) May be associated with Apert syndrome, Saethre–Chotzen, Poland, or other syndromes.

2. Isolated syndactyly (five types):
   a) Long-ring syndactyly is most common.
   b) Look for duplicated phalanges, abnormalities of metacarpals and tarsals.
   c) Autosomal dominant.
   d) Minimal risk of associated anomalies.
3. Poland syndrome:
   a) Simple syndactyly of variable number of fingers.
   b) Short fingers (absent or hypoplastic middle phalanges).
   c) Absent sternocostal head of pectoralis major.
4. Acrocephalosyndactyly
   a) Apert syndrome:
      1. Complete complex syndactyly D2–4 with common nail, progressive interphalangeal synostosis of hands and feet. Medial deviation of great toe and tarsal synostosis.
      2. Craniosynostosis.
      3. Occasional cervical fusions, usually without deformity.
   b) Crouzon syndrome:
      1. Craniosynostosis.
      2. Calcaneocuboid coalition, C-spine fusion.
   c) Many others: Saethre-Chotzen, Carpenter, etc.
5. Congenital constriction bands (Streeter's bands):
   a) Distal (acral) syndactyly with proximal separations.
   b) Thumb rarely involved.
   c) Cutaneous rings or amputations.
   d) May have distal paresis or deformity (clubfoot).
   e) No known Mendelian basis but genetic contribution possible.

5.14.2 Polydactyly

1. Ulnar (postaxial): Frequently isolated, especially in African Americans.
2. Radial (preaxial): More frequently associated with syndromes, especially radial ray defects.
3. Radial clubhand: This is a spectrum that includes hypoplasia to complete absence of preaxial parts. It may be isolated or associated with the following:
   a) Blood dyscrasias:
      1. Fanconi: Anemia to progressive pancytopenia, not present at birth; about a third with renal anomalies; often fatal.
      2. TAR (thrombocytopenia, absent radii) syndrome; neonatal thrombocytopenia, usually improves with time; frequent knee anomalies.
   b) Congenital heart defects:

1. Holt–Oram syndrome: Variable cardiac and preaxial deficiency; most commonly atrial septal defect and hypoplastic thumb.
c) Craniofacial anomalies (Nager syndrome).
d) Congenital scoliosis:
  1. VATER, Goldenhar syndrome (oculo-auriculo-vertebral dysplasia).
  2. Klippel–Feil syndrome.
4. Implications:
  a) Examine previous chest and abdominal films for vertebral anomalies, or take new ones.
  b) Evaluate face, jaw, palate.
  c) Do complete blood and platelet counts.
  d) Ask about feeding (esophageal abnormalities).
  e) Listen to heart, possibly echo.
  f) Evaluate genitourinary system: Urinalysis, possibly echo.
  g) Chromosome analysis if multiple anomalies found outside of the particular syndrome.

5.14.3 Ulnar Clubhand

1. Usually a mild dysgenesis; few frequent associations.
2. May be seen with Cornelia de Lange syndrome.

5.14.4 Amputated Limbs

1. Single: Usually an isolated anomaly but may be associated with idiopathic scoliosis.
2. Congenital ring constriction syndrome.
  a) Nongenetic, variable, rings with grooves in skin, occasionally with lymphatic or vascular impairment.
  b) Transverse amputation with proximal limb normal.
  c) Syndactyly (distal with proximal fenestrations).
  d) Clubfeet.
  e) Craniofacial defects.

5.15 Syndromes with Predominant Spinal Deformity

5.15.1 VA(C)TER(LS)

1. A syndrome or association of unknown etiology, characterized by
  a) Vertebral anomalies.
  b) Anorectal atresia.

c) Cardiac anomalies.

d) *TE* (tracheoesophageal) fistula.

e) *R*enal and radial anomalies (renal atresia, duplication; radial clubhand or preaxial upper-limb hypoplasia).

f) *L*ower-limb abnormalities (duplicated hallux or other anomalies).

g) *S*ingle umbilical artery.

2. Clinical implications: In a patient seen for vertebral anomaly, search for other abnormalities. Obtain renal ultrasound or MRI. Obtain spinal MRI if surgery indicated.

5.15.2 22Q Deletion Syndrome

1. Common chromosomal deletion syndrome encompassing DiGeorge syndrome, velocardiofacial syndrome, conotruncal anomaly face (CTAF) syndrome, and others.

2. Key anomalies include skeletal, palatal, cardiac, and immunologic.

3. Spinal features: Platybasia, occipitalization of the atlas, atlas arch defects, block vertebrae, stenosis, up-turned (swoosh) C2 lamina, thoracolumbar anomalies.

4. Other skeletal anomalies: Equinovarus feet, polydactyly, rib anomalies.

5.15.3 Wildervanck Syndrome

Deafness, Klippel–Feil anomaly, abducens palsy, Chiari malformation.

5.15.4 Goldenhar Syndrome

Also termed oculo-auriculo-vertebral syndrome or hemifacial microsomia. Patients have underdevelopment of the ear, nose, palate and mandible. They often have scoliosis.

5.16 Syndromes Caused by Teratogens

5.16.1 Fetal Alcohol Syndrome

1. Growth disturbance (of both length and weight) through childhood.

2. Central nervous system dysfunction and decreased head size; learning deficit/attention deficit disorder/mental retardation.

3. Dysmorphic face (mild): Small eyes, flat philtrum, thin upper lip.

4. Orthopaedic features:

a) Contractures (elbows, metaphalangeal and interphalangeal joints).
b) Miscellaneous synostoses.
c) Hip dislocations, clubfeet.
d) Congenital cervical fusion (C2–C3 = most).

5.16.2 Fetal Hydantoin Syndrome (from Maternal Use of Phenytoin)

1. Growth retardation: Mild.
2. Mental retardation: Mild.
3. Face: Hypertelorism, cleft lip.
4. Hands: Hypoplasia, absence of phalanges, mostly distal.

5.16.3 Warfarin

Fetal bleeding and teratogenesis.

5.17 Chromosome Abnormalities

5.17.1 Down Syndrome

1. Trisomy, mosaicism, or translocation of chromosome 21.
2. Major findings:
    a) Mental retardation, variable.
    b) Congenital heart defects: arteriovenous communis, ventriculoseptal defect.
    c) Gastrointestinal anomalies.
    d) Short stature.
    e) Leukemia (1%), seizures, diabetes, hypothyroidism: Less frequent.
    f) Orthopaedic:
        1. Delayed walking (1.5–5 years of age).
        2. Ligamentous laxity.
        3. C1–C2 or occiput: C1 laxity: Radiographs at about age 4 and yearly if atlanto-dens interval is greater than 5 mm. Fuse if signs of myelopathy exist.
        4. Scoliosis, idiopathic-like.
        5. Hip dislocations: Acute, subacute, developmental or habitual.
        6. Slipped capital femoral epiphysis.
        7. Perthes disease.
        8. Patellar subluxation or dislocation.
        9. Metatarsus adductus or hallux valgus.

5.17.2 Turner Syndrome

1. Monosomy X.
2. Major findings:
   a) Low birth weight and persistent growth retardation.
   b) Normal intelligence.
   c) Low hairline and webbed neck.
   d) Renal and cardiac anomalies, coarctation.
   e) Absent or hypoplastic gonads.
   f) Orthopaedic:
      1. Genu and cubitus valgus.
      2. Scoliosis, idiopathic.

5.17.3 Noonan Syndrome

1. Turner-like phenotype but normal chromosomes. Defect in *PTPN11* in some cases.
2. Major findings:
   a) Mental retardation.
   b) Hypertelorism, ptosis, downward-slanting eyes.
   c) Increased severity of scoliosis, end-plate changes.
   d) Pulmonary stenosis common.
   e) Thrombocytopenia in some cases.

5.17.4 Klinefelter Syndrome

1. Genetics: 1. 47 XXY.
2. Clinical features:
   a) Asthenic habitus, long legs.
   b) Failure of secondary sexual development.
   c) Scoliosis.
   d) Proximal radioulnar synostosis.

5.17.5 Cri-du-Chat Syndrome

1. Genetics: defect on chromosome 5p.
2. Clinical findings:
   a) Profound mental retardation.
   b) Multiple hand and foot anomalies.
   c) Scoliosis, congenital.

Bibliography

1. Beighton PH, Solomon L, Soskolne CL. Articular mobility in an African population. Ann Rheum Dis. 1973; 32: 413-17
2. Bethem D, Winter RB, Lutter L, et al. Spinal disorders of dwarfism. Review of the literature and report of eighty cases. J Bone Joint Surg Am 1981;63 (9):1412–1425
3. Bitterman AD, Sponseller PD. Marfan syndrome: a clinical update. J Am Acad Orthop Surg 2017;25(9):603–609
4. Goldberg MJ. The Dysmorphic Child: An Orthopaedic Perspective. New York, NY: Raven Press; 1987
5. McKusick V. Online Mendelian Inheritance in Man. Available at: https://www.omim.org/. Accessed June 25, 2018
6. Morcuende JA, Alman BA. Genetic aspects of ortho conditions. In: Weinstein SL, Flynn J, eds. Lovell & Winter's Pediatric Orthopaedics. 7th ed. Philadelphia, PA: J.B. Lippincott; 2014:41–56
7. Sponseller PD. The skeletal dysplasias. In: Weinstein SL, Flynn J, eds. Lovell & Winter's Pediatric Orthopaedics. 7th ed. Philadelphia, PA: J.B. Lippincott; 20014:177–218
8. van Bosse HJ, Saldana RE. Reorientational Proximal Femoral Osteotomies for Arthrogrypotic Hip Contractures. J Bone Joint Surg Am 2017;99(1):55–64

6 Neuromuscular Disorders in Pediatric Orthopaedics

Paul D. Sponseller

6.1 Introduction

This chapter summarizes neuromuscular diseases that affect the skeleton as a result of pathologic conditions of the spinal cord or peripheral nervous system. These diseases may present a fully developed picture or show early subtle findings, such as a mild deviation of gait. The four tables in this chapter organize the neuromuscular diseases according to the location of pathology.

6.2 Evaluation

The elements of evaluation of neuromuscular disease include the following:
1. History: Prenatal, birth (gestation, weight, Apgar scores), developmental (milestones), family; functional deterioration.
2. Physical examination:
   a) Motor strength, tone.
   b) Deep tendon reflexes.
   c) Cranial nerves.
   d) Cerebellar signs.
3. Serum creatine phosphokinase (CPK):
   a) Elevation directly related to amount of muscle necrosis or membrane disorder. Abnormal in Duchenne and Becker muscular dystrophies (> 20 times normal in childhood and early teens), myopathies, or myositis.
   b) Minimal to mild elevation in other dystrophies.
4. Immunocytochemistry: Directly differentiates Duchenne from Becker dystrophies and other conditions. Requires small amount of muscle tissue.
5. DNA mutation analysis: Requires small amount of blood or amniotic fluid, allows prenatal diagnosis.
6. Electromyelography (EMG): Distinguishes myopathic from neuropathic weakness.
   a) Myopathic process: Polyphasic low-voltage signal; fibrillations and sharp waves.
   b) Neuropathic process: Initially, brief biphasic low-voltage fibrillation.
   c) Chronic process: Prolonged polyphasic fibrillation, increased amplitude.
7. Nerve conduction studies:
   a) Abnormally slowed conduction velocities in conditions involving peripheral nerves only.
   b) Normal conduction velocities in spinal muscular atrophy.

c) Normal conduction velocity (> 49 m/s in arms, > 39 m/s in legs) for patients over 5 years of age. Younger children have slower conduction velocity.

8. Muscle biopsy: Biopsy minimally involved muscle in chronic conditions and severely involved muscle in acute conditions. Vastus lateralis used for proximal myopathy should be done only in centers capable of doing special histochemistry.

a) Type I fibers: Oxidative metabolism, slow twitch.

b) Type II fibers: Anaerobic metabolism, fast twitch.

c) Myopathic process:
   1. Necrosis, phagocytosis, and inflammation.
   2. Irregularly sized fibers.
   3. Type I fiber predominance less than 50%.

d) Neuropathic process:
   1. Small group atrophy.
   2. Fiber-type grouping, angular fibers.
   3. Type II fiber predominance greater than 80%.

e) Electron microscopy (glutaraldehyde) is used to differentiate architectural changes within the congenital myopathies.

9. Nerve biopsy:
   a) Sural nerve most commonly biopsied.
   b) Guillain–Barré syndrome: Mononuclear infiltrates and focal acute demyelination.
   c) Hypertrophic neuropathies: Nerve fiber loss, interstitial fibrosis, and "onion bulb" formation.

10. Electrocardiogram and echocardiogram:
   a) Abnormal in Duchenne muscular dystrophy (sinus tachycardia and right ventricular hypertrophy), Friedreich ataxia, and myotonic dystrophy.

11. Genetic testing: available for many disorders; should be ordered by neurologist or neurogeneticist.

6.3 Cerebral Palsy

6.3.1 Definition

Static brain injury or lesion in prenatal, perinatal, or postnatal period (up to 2 years).

6.3.2 Causes

Prematurity, infection, hypoxia, ischemia, embolus, trauma, brain malformation.

6.3.3 Physiologic Types

Pyramidal (spastic), extrapyramidal (dystonic or athetoid), mixed.

6.3.4 Anatomic Types

1. Diplegic: Usually premature. Pyramidal tracts involved; magnetic resonance imaging (MRI) shows periventricular leukomalacia; cognition preserved; legs affected, most distally; equinovalgus feet most common; hips rarely subluxate; scoliosis is rare.
2. Hemiplegic: Focal cortical lesion; risk of seizure; cognition preserved; ipsilateral arm and leg involved. Equinovarus foot is most common; hip and spine involvement is rare. Limb shortening is usually minor.
3. Totally involved (quadriplegic): Usually diffuse cortical problem. Cognition may be affected; problems with spine and trunk balance; respiration and swallowing function affected. Risk of seizure. Hip subluxation, scoliosis, and limb deformities are common.
4. Other types: Monoplegia, asymmetric diplegia.

6.3.5 Gross Motor Functional Classification System (▶ Fig. 6.1; ▶ Fig. 6.2)

1. Level I: Walks without restrictions, but speed and coordination are impaired.
2. Level II: Walks indoors and outdoors and climbs stairs using railing; difficulty with uneven surfaces.
3. Level III: Uses crutches to walk. Propels own manual wheelchair.
4. Level IV: Walks short distance with walker; uses wheelchair more.
5. Level V: Trunk and all extremities are involved. No independent mobility.
Subclassification based on axial impairment: additional 0.1 for each of the following: nonverbal status, seizure disorder, G-tube, tracheostomy.

6.3.6 Hip Subluxation Rating

Reimer migration index (MI) is the percentage of femoral head lateral to the Perkin line (A/B below); quantitates MI (▶ Fig. 6.3).

6.3.7 Treatment

1. Physical therapy.
2. Mobility aids (orthoses, crutches, walker, and wheelchair).
3. Oral medications for spasticity, dystonia.
4. Botulinum toxin for temporary tone management.

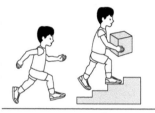

GMFCS Level I

Children walk indoors and outdoors and climb stairs without limitation. Children perform gross motor skills including running and jumping, but speed, balance and coordination are impaired.

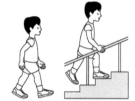

GMFCS Level II

Children walk indoors and outdoors and climb stairs holding onto a railing but experience limitations walking on uneven surfaces and inclines and walking in crowds or confined spaces.

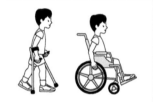

GMFCS Level III

Children walk indoors or outdoors on a level surface with an assistive mobility device. Children may climb stairs holding onto a railing. Children may propel a wheelchair manually or are transported when traveling for long distances or outdoors on uneven terrain.

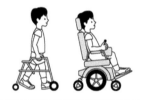

GMFCS Level IV

Children may continue to walk for short distances on a walker or rely more on wheeled mobility at home and school and in the community.

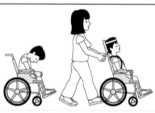

GMFCS Level V

Physical impairment restricts voluntary control of movement and the ability to maintain antigravity head and trunk postures. All areas of motor function are limited. Children have no means of independent mobility and are transported.

Fig. 6.1 Gross motor functional classification system. (Used with permission from Graham HK. Classifying cerebral palsy. J Pediatr Orthop 2005;25(1):128 (Fig. 1).)

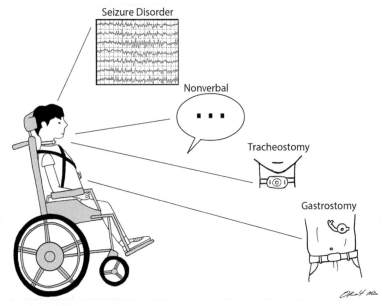

Fig. 6.2 Subclassification of GMFCS5 based on additional axial neuro impairments predicts function and complications.

5. Selective dorsal rhizotomy for lower-extremity spasticity.
6. Intrathecal pump for generalized spasticity.
7. Orthopaedic muscle lengthening and transfer.
8. Osteotomies for bony deformity.
9. Arthrodesis of spine or feet if collapse impairs function.

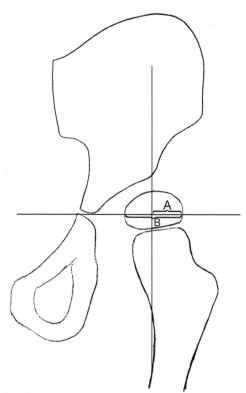

Fig. 6.3 The percentage of femoral head lateral to the Perkin line (A/B) quantitates the Reimer migration index.

6.4 Disorders of Spinal Cord Peripheral Nerves and Muscles

6.4.1 Anterior Horn Cell Diseases (▶ Table 6.1)

Table 6.1 Anterior horn cell disorders

Disease	Age at diagnosis	Inheritance pattern	Life expectancy	Signs	Orthopaedic manifestations	Laboratories
Polio	Variable	None (infectious)	Related to level of involvement	Asymmetric flaccid paralysis, asymmetric or absent DTR	Contractures, scoliosis	Depends on phase of illness
Spinal muscular atrophy						
Type I or Werdnig–Hoffman	Birth to 6 mo	Autosomal recessive gene defect on 5q-SMN gene	Most die in infancy	Marked general weakness, no head control, absent DTR normal sensation	Fractures	
Type II	6–12 mo	Autosomal recessive gene defect on 5q	Early to mid-adulthood	Normal until ~6 mo, independent head control in sitting position, never ambulate	Hip subluxation, scoliosis, contracture	EMG: high-amplitude polyphasic NCS: widespread fascicular pattern of denervation
Type III Kugelberg–Welander	1–2 y	Autosomal recessive gene defect on 5q	Over 45 y	Normal until ~1 y, ambulate until 2nd decade, then wheelchair, never can run or climb stairs	Kyphosis, scoliosis	DNA test for SMN, same as type II

Abbreviations: DTR, deep tendon reflex; EMG, electromyelography; NCS, nerve conduction study.

6.4.2 Neuropathies (▶ Table 6.2)

Table 6.2 Neuropathies

Disease	Age of diagnosis	Inheritance pattern	Life expectancy	Signs	Orthopaedic manifestations	Laboratories
Guillain–Barré syndrome	Variable	None; postviral infection	~ 5% mortality	Ascending pain, paresthesia, and weakness	Contractures	↑ CSF protein
Friedreich ataxia (spinocerebellar degeneration)	Before 10 y	Autosomal dominant chromosome 9 defect	<40 y	Wide-based gait weakness, tremor, nystagmus, uses wheelchair by age 30; areflexia cardiomyopathy	Pas cavus, scoliosis, ataxia, speech disorder	↓ ↓ Sensory and ↓ motor conduction velocity
Hereditary motor and sensory neuropathies						
Type I: Demyelinating form of Charcot–Marie–Tooth	Second decade of life	Autosomal dominant	Normal	Foot deformity, intrinsic wasting, absent reflexes, length-dependent weakness, sensory ↓	Equinocavovarus clawing, gait abnormality, hip dysplasia, scoliosis (10%)	↓ Motor conduction velocity
Type II or Charcot–Marie–Tooth disease (axonal form)	Wide variation	Autosomal dominant	Normal	"Stork legs," foot deformity, distal weakness	Cavus foot deformities, occasional UE intrinsic weakness, gait abnormality	Normal or slight ↓ motor conduction velocity
Type III or Dejerine–Sottas disease	Infancy to early childhood	Autosomal recessive	Wide variation	Same as CMT but more severe	Cavus foot, scoliosis	↓ ↓ Motor conduction velocity, ↑ CSF protein

Abbreviations: CMT, Charcot-Marie-Tooth disease; CSF, cerebrospinal fluid.

175

6.4.3 Muscular Dystrophies (▶ Table 6.3)

Table 6.3 Muscular dystrophies

Disease	Age at diagnosis	Inheritance pattern	Abnormal gene	Life expectancy	Signs	Orthopaedic manifestations	Laboratories
DMD	2–6 y	X-linked recessive (have new mutation)	Xp21	~20–30 y	Late walker, calf pseudohypertrophy, Meryon and Gower signs, mild mental retardation	Contractures: equinovarus, knee flexion, hip flexion–abduction, wheelchair dependence, scoliosis	↑↑ CK, ↓↓ dystrophin
Becker muscular dystrophy	Childhood	X-linked recessive	Xp21	Adulthood	Weakness, pseudohypertrophy	Contractures, wheelchair dependence late	↑CK, ↓dystrophin
Limb–Girdle dystrophy	2nd to 3rd decades of life	Autosomal recessive and dominant forms	Many	Wide range	Weakness of pelvic or shoulder-girdle muscles	Similar to DMD, milder	↑CK, normal dystrophin
Fascioscapulohumeral dystrophy	2nd decade of life	Autosomal dominant	4q	Normal	Facial and shoulder-girdle weakness, expressionless face	Scapular winging contractures	Mild ↑ CPK, normal dystrophin
Emery–Dreifuss dystrophy	2–4 y	X-linked recessive	Xq28	Mid-adult	Muscle weakness, AV block	Toe-walking, elbow flexion contractures neck extension	CK min ↑ normal dystrophin
Congenital myopathies							
Nemaline-body myopathy	Variable	Sarcomere proteins		Variable		Scoliosis proximal weakness	
Central core myopathy	Infancy				Nonprogressive	Kyphoscoliosis equinovarus feet	
Centronuclear myopathy		X-linked recessive	Xq28			DDH	

Abbreviations: AV, arteriovenous; CK, creatine kinase; CPK, creatine phosphokinase; DDH, developmental dysplasia of the hip; DMD, Duchenne muscular dystrophy.

6.4.4 Myotonic Disorders (▶ Table 6.4)

Table 6.4 Myotonic disorders

Disease	Age of diagnosis	Inheritance pattern	Abnormal gene	Life expectancy	Signs
Myotonia congenita	0–10 y	Autosomal dominant		Normal	Myotonia with initial movement. General muscular hypertrophy. Dilantin and procainamide can decrease myotonia
Paramyotonia congenita	Childhood	Autosomal dominant		Normal	Cold-induced episodes of paradoxical myotonia and flaccid paresis associated with K$^+$ abnormalities treated with quinine or ion exchange resins
Myotonic dystrophy	2nd to 3rd decades of life	Autosomal dominant	CTG expansion	Decreased	Progressive weakness begins distally. Gonadal atrophy, cataracts, heart disease, and mental defects associated. Develop C spine subluxation and wheelchair dependency
Congenital myotonic dystrophy	Infancy	Autosomal dominant	Large CTG expansion	Normal	Hypotonia, difficulty swallowing, and expressionless faces. Develop clubfeet, contractures and dislocated hips, mental defects, and lenticular opacities associated. EMG: pathognomonic "dive bomber" pattern disease becomes more severe with second-generation equinovarus feet

Abbreviations: EMG, electromyelography; CTG, cytosine, thymine, guanine.

6.4.5 Spina Bifida

1. Classification: Myelomeningocele or lipomeningocele.
2. Associated abnormalities: Congenital spine deformity, Sprengel deformity, Chiari malformation, tethered cord, neurogenic bladder. High risk of latex allergy.
3. Motor classification and implications:

   a) Thoracic/high lumbar: Minimal ambulation; highest risk of associated deformities.

   b) Midlumbar: May ambulate but stop at maturity; highest risk of hip dislocation.

   c) Low lumbar (quadriceps and hamstrings function): Moderate walking with limp.

   d) Sacral: Near-normal walking.
4. Treatment:

   a) Physical therapy to optimize strength and motion; match equipment to functional level.

   b) Monitor for tethered cord (increasing weakness, back pain, unexpected scoliosis).

   c) Brace feet, ankles, and knees if able to improve function.

   d) Treat hip dislocations only if L5 level or below.

   e) Release contractures only if functionally significant.

   f) Treat clubfeet aggressively with casts, braces, and surgery as needed.

   g) Monitor for potential skin pressure areas and prevent with bracing or surgery.

   h) Avoid latex.

   i) Optimize vitamin D intake.

   j) Recognize fractures presenting as warm, swollen limb in the absence of trauma.

Bibliography

1. Graham HK. Classifying cerebral palsy. J Pediatr Orthop 2005;25(1):127–128
2. Jain A, Sponseller PD, Shah SA, et al; Harms Study Group. Subclassification of GMFCS Level-5 cerebral palsy as a predictor of complications and health-related quality of life after spinal arthrodesis. J Bone Joint Surg Am 2016;98 (21):1821–1828
3. Shapiro F, Specht L. The diagnosis and orthopaedic treatment of inherited muscular diseases of childhood. J Bone Joint Surg Am 1993;75(3):439–454
4. Shapiro F, Specht L. The diagnosis and orthopaedic treatment of childhood spinal muscular atrophy, peripheral neuropathy, Friedreich ataxia, and arthrogryposis. J Bone Joint Surg Am 1993;75(11):1699–1714

7 Pediatric Trauma

Paul D. Sponseller and Matthew J. Hadad

7.1 Introduction

This chapter begins with a presentation of the unique considerations in pediatric trauma, followed by a systematic, proximal-to-distal presentation of the principles and algorithms for the management of pediatric orthopaedic trauma. Common diaphyseal fractures are not covered if there are no unique pediatric features. References are provided at the end of each section for further information.

7.2 Basic Principles

7.2.1 Differences in Anatomy

1. Periosteum:
   a) Thicker and stronger in children.
   b) Often intact on the compressed side of fractures; use as hinge in reduction.
2. Elastic bones:
   a) Torus/buckle fractures: Bulging of the cortex after axial loading force.
   b) Greenstick fractures: Incomplete fracture on one side of diaphysis.
   c) Bowing fracture: Bending of bone without visible fracture or cortical injury.

7.2.2 Physeal Fractures Classification

1. There are several classification systems, but the most commonly used is still that of Salter and Harris. The systems' goals are to (1) facilitate communication, (2) predict the risk of growth disturbance, and (3) determine treatment.
2. The classifications provide information on:
   a) Physeal alignment.
   b) Articular alignment.
   c) Stability and risk of displacement.
3. Physeal damage can occur from:
   a) Step off at the level of the physis, with bar formation.
   b) Damage to and death of physeal cells.
   c) Ischemia of the physis if severe soft-tissue damage occurs.
4. The classifications are usually predictive of the risk of growth disturbance. Salter I and II fractures are typically at low risk of growth disturbance because the growth plate is not traversed by the fracture. However, there

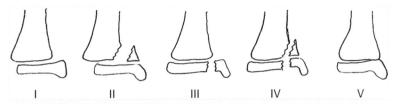

Fig. 7.1 Salter–Harris classification of physeal injuries.

are some notable exceptions because damage may occur to the physis but not be visible on plain films. This is most common in the distal femur and the distal tibia, where there is a high risk of growth disturbance even in the "benign" fracture types such as Salter I and II. This may be due to complex physeal anatomy as well as compressive forces involved. By contrast, there is a low risk of growth plate damage in Salter I and II fractures of the distal radius and ulna and the proximal humerus.

5. Salter–Harris classification: The most widely used (▶ Fig. 7.1). Note that type V fractures are rarely, if ever, seen.
6. Peterson classification: Recognizes a broader spectrum of injuries.

7.2.3 Management of the Polytrauma Patient

Definition: The polytrauma patient is a patient with more than one organ system injured or more than one component injured within one organ system.

1. Laboratory studies: Complete blood cell count, type and cross, urinalysis, blood urea nitrogen, creatinine, amylase, electrolytes.
2. Indications for radiographic studies:
   a) Cervical, thoracic, lumbar spine:
      1. Tender.
      2. Unconscious or heavily sedated.
      3. Neurologically abnormal.
   b) Pelvis:
      1. Tender.
      2. Unconscious.
      3. Hematuria present.
   c) Skull:
      1. Head trauma and loss of consciousness for longer than 5 minutes, hematoma.
      2. Skull depression.
      3. Focal neurologic signs.
      4. Cerebrospinal fluid from nose or middle ear.
      5. Blood in middle ear.

d) Computed tomography (CT) of the head:
 1. Glasgow Coma Scale score less than 8.
 2. Focal neurologic signs.
 3. CT of the abdomen.
 4. Shock.
 5. Severe head injury.
 6. Abnormal abdominal examination.

7.2.4 Evaluation of Patient

1. Primary survey: To detect most urgent priorities ("ABCDE").
   - A—Airway.
   - B—Breathing (ventilation).
   - C—Circulation (hemorrhage).
   - D—Disability (neurologic status).
   - E—Exposure (temperature).
2. Secondary survey:
   a) Complete physical examination.
   b) History of event.
   c) Medical history.
   d) Laboratory and radiographic results.
   e) Reevaluation and stabilization.
3. Normal vital signs for children (▶ Table 7.1).
4. Glasgow Coma Scale (▶ Table 7.2).

Table 7.1 Normal vital signs by age

Age	Pulse (beats/min)	Respirations (per min)	Blood pressure (mm Hg, systolic / diastolic)
1–6 mo	130 ± 45	30–40	80/46
6–12 mo	114 ± 40	24–30	95/65
1–2 y	110 ± 40	20–30	99/65
2–6 y	105 ± 35	20–25	100/60
6–12 y	95 ± 30	16–20	110/60
12 y	80 ± 25	12–16	120/60

Table 7.2 The Glasgow Coma Scale

Response	Score
Eye opening	
• None	1
• To pain	2
• To voice	3
• Spontaneous	4
Verbal	
• None	1
• Incomprehensible	2
• Inappropriate	3
• Disoriented	4
• Oriented	5
Motor	
• None	1
• Decerebrate	2
• Decorticate	3
• Withdraws from pain	4
• Localizes to pain	5
• Obeys commands	6
Total	**Up to 15 points**

7.2.5 Adjuncts in Management

1. Intracranial pressure measurement indications:
   a) Glasgow Coma Scale less than 5, or less than 8 if shock is present.
   b) CT scan showing mass or shift.
   c) Progressive neurologic deterioration.
2. Parenteral nutrition: indicated in polytrauma patient if enteral feeding not expected within 24 hours.
3. Repeat physical examination: Should be performed at 24 and 48 hours because of the incidence of missed injuries (bone scan is an alternative).
4. Indications for deep venous thrombosis prophylaxis in polytrauma:
   a) Oral contraceptive use.
   b) Vascular injury.
   c) Sickle cell anemia.
   d) Prolonged immobility in older adolescents.

7.3 Pediatric Shoulder Injuries

7.3.1 Principles

1. The proximal humeral physis is one of the most active in the skeleton, contributing 80% of the length of the humerus: therefore, it has tremendous remodeling potential.
2. Ossification:
    a) Begins at 6 months in proximal humeral epiphysis, and growth ceases at 15 years in girls and 18 years in boys.
    b) Ossific center for greater tuberosity appears at age 1; medial clavicle physis closes at around 23 years.

7.3.2 Birth Fractures

1. Risk factors:
    a) Difficult delivery.
    b) Large size.
    c) Breech presentation.
2. Presentation:
    a) "Pseudoparalysis"—limb moves little.
    b) Rule out sepsis, brachial plexus injury.
3. Diagnosis: Plain radiographs or ultrasound.
4. Treatment: Gently immobilize the arm to the chest using an Ace wrap.

7.3.3 Proximal Humeral Fractures

1. Background:
    a) Age-based patterns: Preadolescent usually has fracture of metaphyseal region; adolescent, physeal fracture; Salter I or II.
    b) Mechanism: Axial load or abduction; external rotation.
    c) Muscle insertions with respect to physis: Internal and external rotators all on proximal fragment; deltoid and pectoralis, distal fragment displaces anteriorly and medially.
2. Criteria for acceptable alignment:
    a) Child younger than 12 years: Virtually any alignment is acceptable.
    b) Child older than 12 years: Shortening or overlap less than 3 cm.
    c) Angulation less than 45 degrees.
3. Classification of displacement (pediatric):
    a) Neer and Horowitz:
        • I: Less than 5 mm translation.
        • II: 5 mm to 33%.
        • III: 33 to 66%.
        • IV: Greater than 66% (most are grade IV).

Translation itself is not a problem. *Note:* Appearance on emergency department film is not the same as the appearance later. Angulation usually improves.

1. Treatment methods:
   a) Sling.
   b) Traction.
   c) Shoulder spica.
   d) Abduction brace.
   e) Internal fixation.
2. General recommendations:
   a) If alignment is acceptable, swing or hang cast.
   b) Reduce and pin if < 2 years of growth remaining and > 45 degrees malalignment.
   c) Additionally, consider open reduction and internal fixation (ORIF) if:
      1. Severe head injury with spasticity.
      2. Polytrauma: To facilitate management.
      3. Vascular injury.
      4. Tenting skin: Risk of breakdown.
3. Fracture through unicameral bone cyst (UBC):
   a) Common cause of proximal humerus fracture in child.
   b) Differential diagnosis:
      1. Eosinophilic granuloma.
      2. Aneurysmal bone cyst (ABC).
      3. Fibrous dysplasia.
      4. Fibrous cortical defect.
   c) Treatment of UBC:
      1. Sling to heal fracture: 4 to 6 weeks.
      2. Cyst regresses about 20% of time.
      3. Assess and discuss the risk of refracture with family: depends mainly on cortical thickness.
      4. Inject with methylprednisolone or bone graft if (a) persistently thin cortex; (b) high desired activity level; (c) family prefers active treatment.
      5. May need several injections.

7.3.4 Sternoclavicular Injuries

Background

1. Medial clavicle is last epiphysis to appear and to close (< 23 years old), providing 80% of clavicle growth.
2. Medial fracture: Usually Salter–Harris I or II physeal separation; epiphysis hard to visualize.

3. Diaphyseal fracture: More common, middle one-third of clavicle.
4. Mechanism: Fall on outstretched arm or other lateral force on shoulder girdle.

Treatment

1. Medial fracture:
   a) CT often necessary to identify.
   b) Anterior or superior displacement: usually no reduction attempted.
   c) Posterior displacement: reduce if significant dysphagia or pulmonary issues.
2. Diaphyseal fracture:
   a) Reduction generally not attempted in children or adolescents.
   b) Treat only if *significant* displacement or evidence of:
      1. Venous congestion.
      2. Decreased pulse.
      3. Difficulty breathing, swallowing.
      4. Sensation of choking.
3. Operative treatment, if indicated:
   a) Closed reduction: May use towel clips.
   b) Internal fixation: use sutures if unstable.
4. Reassure family that a bump will occur and gradually shrink at the site of remodeling.

Bibliography

1. Bae DS, Kocher MS, Waters PM, Micheli LM, Griffey M, Dichtel L. Chronic recurrent anterior sternoclavicular joint instability: results of surgical management. J Pediatr Orthop 2006;26(1):71–74
2. Baxter MP, Willey JJ. Fractures of the proximal humeral epiphysis. Their influence on humeral growth. J Bone Joint Surg Br 1986;68(4):570573
3. Skaggs DL, Frick S. Management of fractures. In: Morrissy RT, Weinstein SL, Flynn JM, eds. Lovelland Winter's Pediatric Orthopaedics. 7th ed. Philadelphia, PA: Lippincott Williams & Wilkins; 20014:1694–1773

7.4 Pediatric Elbow Injuries

7.4.1 Supracondylar Humerus Fracture

Background and classification:

1. Direction of displacement:

    a) 95% are due to hyperextension; periosteal hinge will be posterior.

    b) 5% are due to flexion; periosteal hinge will be anterior.

2. Degree of displacement (Gartland classification):

    a) Type I: Undisplaced.

    b) Type II: Hinged/greenstick fracture:

       1. IIa: Not rotated.

       2. IIb: Rotated.

    c) Type III: Completely displaced with intact periosteal hinge.

    d) Type IV: Multidirectionally unstable without periosteal hinge.

7.4.2 Principle

Type III fractures have an appreciable incidence of nerve and artery damage with little intrinsic stability. Pretreatment neurovascular exam is essential, which includes the following:

1. Median nerve: Check active palmar flexion.

2. Anterior interosseous nerve: Distal interphalangeal (DIP) flexion of index finger and thumb.

3. Posterior interosseous nerve: Dorsiflexion of the metacarpophalangeal joints.

4. Ulnar nerve: Flexion of the fifth finger distal interphalangeal joint or crossing of the index and second fingers (▶ Fig. 7.2).

7.4.3 Treatment

1. Type II: Check varus valgus and consider reduction if the Baumann angle is greater than 5 to 10 degrees off normal.

2. Type III: Percutaneous pin fixation best (▶ Fig. 7.3): One medial and lateral or two lateral pins. Both pins should start distal to the fracture site with longitudinal traction and slight flexion. The lateral pin should engage a portion of the capitellum, and the medial pin should be slightly medial and anterior on the epicondyle to avoid the ulnar nerve (▶ Fig. 7.4). Make a small incision to clear a tract. If two lateral pins are used, one should cross the lateral third of the fracture, and one should cross the central third of the fracture (▶ Fig. 7.5).

3. If anatomic closed reduction is not possible, perform open reduction. Check alignment of the fracture using the Baumann angle (▶ Fig. 7.6a); normal is

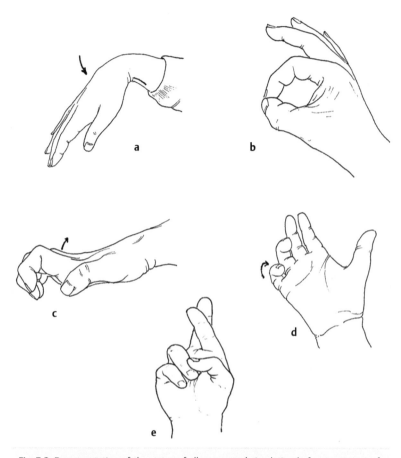

Fig. 7.2 Documentation of the status of all nerves and circulation before treatment of supracondylar humerus fractures. This involves (a) checking active palmar flexion (median nerve); (b) flexion of distal interphalangeal joints of the index finger and thumb-anterior interosseous nerve; (c) dorsiflexion of the metacarpophalangeal joints—posterior interosseous nerve; (d) flexion of the fifth finger distal interphalangeal joint; or (e) crossing of index and second fingers—ulnar nerve.

72 ± 4 degrees. Also check the anterior humeral line (▶ Fig. 7.6b), which should intersect the anterior one-third to one-half of the capitellum.

4. Aftercare: May begin protected range of motion at around 3 weeks with temporary splint removal. Remove pins at 6 weeks.

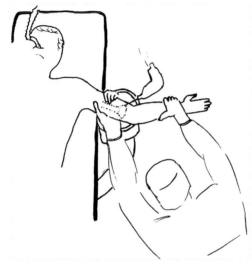

Fig. 7.3 One technique of closed reduction and percutaneous pinning. Longitudinal traction is applied in slight flexion to correct angulation and yet allow visualization. Fluoroscopy receiver serves as platform.

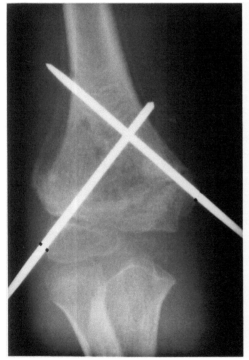

Fig. 7.4 Desired pin placement for medial and lateral pin technique.

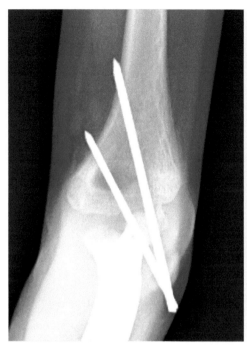

Fig. 7.5 Lateral pin fixation for type III supracondylar humerus fractures.

7.4.4 Nerve Injury

1. Frequency: Radial > anterior interosseous > ulnar > median.
2. Treatment: If deficit is present before reduction, then it is probably a neuropraxia resulting from the injury; proceed with closed reduction. If no return by 5 months after injury, then obtain electromyelogram; explore and perform neurolysis if no recovery.

7.4.5 Arterial Insufficiency

1. Reduce fracture; do not hyperflex:
   a) If perfusion returns, pin fracture.
   b) If perfusion does not return, perform an open exploration through an anterior Henry approach.
   c) If artery is entrapped, release and watch.
   d) If in spasm, use lidocaine.
   e) If an intimal tear occurs, repair.
   f) If transected, vein graft.

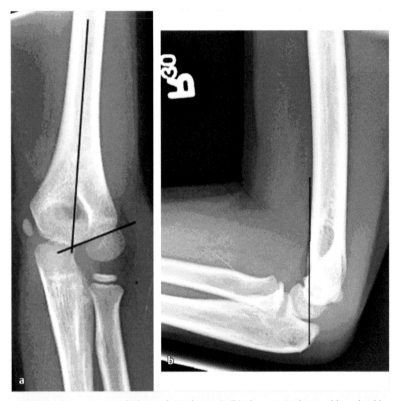

Fig. 7.6 **(a)** Baumann angle (normal, 72 degrees). **(b)** The anterior humeral line should intersect anterior or middle third of capitellum.

2. Measure compartment pressures after reperfusion and perform fasciotomy if needed.

7.4.6 Lateral Condyle Fracture

1. Background:
   a) Mechanism: fall onto outstretched hand.
   b) Collateral vascular supply to the capitellum and lateral trochlea mostly enters posteriorly.
   c) Fracture may occur with varus or valgus force.

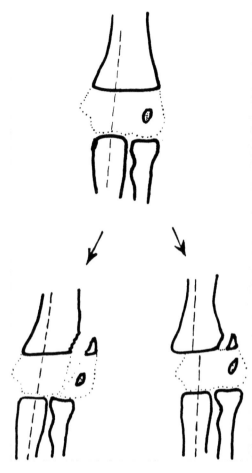

Fig. 7.7 Differentiation of lateral condyle from distal humeral physeal fracture. In the latter, displacement of the entire forearm follows the metaphyseal fragment. In minimally displaced fractures, physical examination, ultrasound, arthrogram, or MRI may be helpful. The top illustration shows normal alignment of ulna and humerus. (Lower left) Alignment maintained in lateral condyle fracture. (Lower right) Alignment is lost in distal humeral Salter II physeal fractures.

   d) Distinguish this injury from a transphyseal separation by lack of swelling and tenderness medially and by alignment of the humerus with the forearm (▶ Fig. 7.7); ultrasound may help.

   e) Internal oblique radiograph shows the fracture best.

2. Principles and significance:

   a) Lateral condyle fracture is one of the few pediatric fractures in which nonunion and avascular necrosis are not rare.

   b) Cast is rarely able to maintain reduction of a displaced lateral condyle.

3. Jakob classification:

   a) Type I: < 2 mm displacement, undisplaced.

b) Type II: > 2 mm displacement, hinged.

c) Type III: > 2 mm displacement, translated.

4. Treatment:

    a) Type I: Splint in 90 to 100 degrees of flexion; pronation: recheck at 5 and 10 days (ORIF if further displacement).

    b) Type II or III, or if follow-up is unreliable: Attempt closed reduction (optional):

        1. Avoid posterior dissection; visualize reduction anteriorly.

        2. Internal fixation: Two divergent pins preferred.

        3. May cross physis if needed.

        4. May use screw; remove later.

        5. Usually remove pins and splint at 6 to 8 weeks.

    c) Fiberglass allows best visualization of fracture.

    d) Late presentation (displaced and ununited longer than 6 weeks):

        1. Approach anteriorly with graft and rigid fixation if in good position (early). Operate only for lateral instability symptoms if after 3 weeks. Avoid excessive dissection.

        2. Valgus osteotomy if significant deformity exists.

        3. Ulnar nerve anterior transposition if deformity is increasing.

7.4.7 Medial Epicondyle Fractures

1. Background:

    a) Medial epicondyle begins to ossify at 4 to 6 years; fuses at around 15 years of age.

    b) Fracture most common in ages 9 to 12 years.

    c) Significance of this fracture:

        1. Medial collateral ligament of ulna attaches to the base of the epicondyle.

        2. Entrapped medial epicondyle may be missed.

        3. Look for medial condylar extension.

2. Treatment:

    a) Principle: Displacement is well tolerated unless forceful loading is anticipated.

    b) Indications for ORIF:

        1. Epicondyle in joint despite attempt at manipulation.

        2. High valgus stresses anticipated (dominant arm of throwing athlete, etc.) in patient with displaced epicondyle. "Stress test" in 15 degrees of flexion may be of interest, but most are unstable acutely; no specific guidelines for interpretation of this test exist.

    c) Technique of ORIF: Exposure is easier in prone position. May use screw or percutaneous pin. Ulnar nerve transposition is not recommended in most cases.

d) Indications for closed reduction: All cases not meeting the preceding criteria for ORIF, including the following special cases:
  1. Acute ulnar neuropathy: Likely to resolve with time; not a specific indication for ORIF or ulnar nerve transposition.
  2. Displacement greater than 5 mm but not intra-articular.
  3. Epicondyle fracture with elbow dislocation.
e) Technique of closed reduction: Extend elbow, wrist, and fingers simultaneously with slight valgus.

7.4.8 Elbow Dislocations

1. Background:
   a) Dislocation without fracture is more common in older children. In young children, physis is weaker than ligaments.
   b) Before skeletal maturity, about 60% have associated fracture:
      1. Medial epicondyle.
      2. Proximal radius.
      3. Coronoid.
      4. Olecranon.
      5. Osteochondral coronoid flap.
   c) *Open* dislocations have a high incidence of arterial injury.
2. Treatment:
   a) Carefully examine for associated fractures, especially of radial head or lateral condyle.
   b) Closed reduction with sedation or anesthesia is successful in most cases.
   c) Instruct parent in vascular examination.
   d) Splint for 2 to 3 weeks.
   e) Follow-up to rule out posterolateral instability.
   f) If dislocation is missed for longer than 1 week, open reduction is needed.

7.4.9 Nursemaid Elbow (Annular Ligament Entrapment)

1. Caused by longitudinal traction in child 1 to 4 years old.
2. Elbow held slightly flexed, pronated, and guarded.
3. Radiographs are normal.
4. Treatment: Flex and supinate (▶ Fig. 7.8); immobilization is usually not needed.

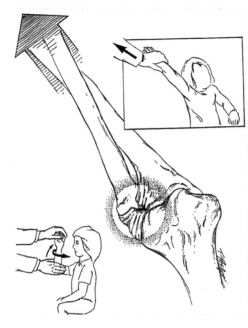

Fig. 7.8 Nursemaid's elbow. Mechanism is traction and pronation. Reduction is by flexion and supination. (Used with permission from Sponseller PD. Bone, joint, and muscle. In: Oski FA, ed. Principles and Practice of Pediatrics. 2nd ed. Philadelphia, PA: J.B. Lippincott; 1994:1037 (Fig. 38–25).)

7.4.10 Radial Head and Neck Fractures

Background

1. Secondary ossification center appears around 4 to 5 years.
2. Much of radial neck is intracapsular.

Wilkins Classification: Consider Location and Mechanism

1. Group 1: Primary displacement of *radial head*:
   a) Valgus fractures:
      1. Type A: Salter I and II.
      2. Type B: Salter IV.
      3. Type C: Metaphyseal fractures without physeal fracture.
   b) Fractures with elbow dislocation:
      1. Type D: Reduction injuries.
      2. Type E: Dislocation injuries.
2. Group 2: Primary dislocation of *radial neck*:
   a) Angular injuries: associated with proximal ulnar fracture (Monteggia).
   b) Torsional injuries.

3. **Group 3**: Stress injuries:
   a) Osteochondritis of the radial head.
   b) Physeal injuries with neck angulation.

Treatment Guidelines

1. More than 30 degrees of angulation: Accept posterior splint or long-arm cast, begin range of motion in 1 to 2 weeks.
2. 30 to 45 degrees of angulation: Manipulate but accept closed result.
3. More than 45 degrees (approximately) or translocated: Manipulate but require ORIF if unsuccessful.

Manipulation Techniques (with Patient under Anesthesia)

1. Traction in extension (Patterson manipulative technique):
   a) Use fluoroscopy to profile fracture.
   b) Press on displaced fragment.
   c) Apply varus stress to forearm.
2. Flexion-pronation technique:
   a) Flex elbow 90 degrees.
   b) Rotate forearm from full.
   c) Supination to pronation while applying pressure anteriorly to radial head.
3. Percutaneous K-wire leverage:
   a) Elbow in extension.
   b) Use fluoroscopy.
   c) Pin starts proximally in the "corner" of the radial head, behind the posterior interosseous nerve.
4. Métaizeau technique: 2.0 to 2.5 mm intramedullary rod from the distal radial metaphysis advanced retrograde into the epiphysis to obtain or maintain reduction.

Maintaining Reduction

1. Flexion to 90 degrees if stable.
2. For unstable fractures, prefer oblique K wire from proximal to distal fragment. Protect with posterior splint.

7.4.11 Monteggia Fracture Dislocation

1. Definition: Fracture of the proximal or middle third of the ulna with dislocation of the radial head.

2. Principle: Radial head dislocates in the direction in which a line through the distal ulnar fragment is pointing. Even a slight ulnar bend may be a sign of radial head subluxation (▶ Fig. 7.9).
3. Bado classification (based on the direction of *radial head* dislocation):
   a) Type I: Anterior dislocation (▶ Fig. 7.10).
   b) Type II: Posterior dislocation.
   c) Type III: Lateral dislocation.
   d) Type IV: Anterior dislocation with fracture of proximal third of the radius.

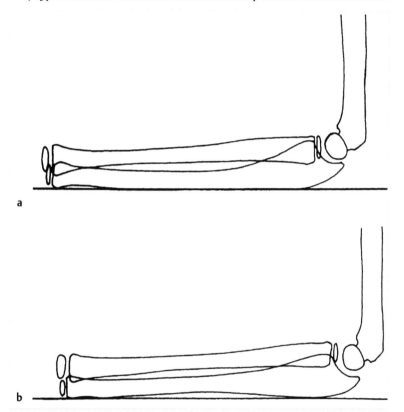

Fig. 7.9 Ulnar bow sign. (**a**) Maximum deviation of the elbow cortex from a straight line should be 1 mm. (**b**) If greater, it should suggest plastic deformation of the ulna, and radial head subluxation is possible. (Used with permission from Lincoln TL, Mubarak SJ. "Isolated" traumatic radial-head dislocation. J Pediatr Orthop 1994;14(4):455 (Fig. 1AB).)

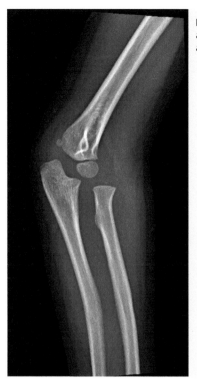

Fig. 7.10 Bado type I Monteggia with anterior dislocation of radial head and apex-anterior ulnar greenstick fracture.

4. Treatment:
   a) Reduction mechanism used to reduce the ulnar fracture, with supination added for anterior and lateral types of dislocation. The cast varies by type (▸ Fig. 7.11):
      1. Type 1: Flexion and supination.
      2. Type 2: Full extension and supination.
      3. Type 3: Full extension and supination with valgus mold over radial head.
   b) Failure to achieve or maintain radial head reduction: Intramedullary pinning or plating of ulna.
   c) If this does not reduce the radial head, then openly reduce it.
5. Late-presenting Monteggia fracture dislocation can be operatively reduced up to several years after injury. Correct the ulnar bow and reconstruct the annular ligament (Bell Tawse procedure).

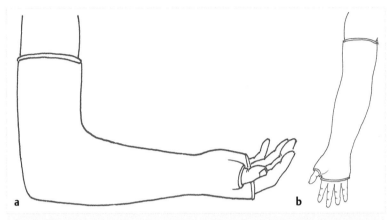

Fig. 7.11 (**a**) Bado type I (anterior) Monteggia fractures should be reduced and immobilized with the elbow in flexion and supination. (**b**) Bado type II (posterior) and III (lateral) Monteggia fractures are reduced and immobilized with the elbow in extension and supination, with a valgus mold over the radial head.

Bibliography

General
1. Wilkins KE. Elbow fractures. In: Wilkins KE, Beaty JH, eds. Fractures in Children. Philadelphia, PA: Lippincott; 2006

Supracondylar Fractures
1. Culp RW, Osterman AL, Davidson RS, Skirven T, Bora FW Jr. Neural injuries associated with supracondylar fractures of the humerus in children. J Bone Joint Surg Am 1990;72(8):1211–1215
2. Omid R, Choi PD, Skaggs DL. Supracondylar humeral fractures in children. J Bone Joint Surg Am 2008;90(5):1121–1132
3. Pirone AM, Graham HK, Krajbich JI. Management of displaced extension-type supracondylar fractures of the humerus in children. J Bone Joint Surg Am 1988;70(5):641–650
4. Skaggs DL, Cluck MW, Mostofi A, Flynn JM, Kay RM. Lateral-entry pin fixation in the management of supracondylar fractures in children. J Bone Joint Surg Am 2004;86-A(4):702–707

Lateral Condyle Fracture
1. Badelon O, Bensahel H, Mazda K, Vie P. Lateral humeral condylar fractures in children: a report of 47 cases. J Pediatr Orthop 1988;8(1):31–34

2. Flynn JC. Nonunion of slightly displaced fractures of the lateral humeral condyle in children: an update. J Pediatr Orthop 1989;9(6):691–696
3. Song KS, Kang CH, Min BW, Bae KC, Cho CH. Internal oblique radiographs for diagnosis of nondisplaced or minimally displaced lateral condylar fractures of the humerus in children. J Bone Joint Surg Am 2007;89(1):58–63
4. Stein BE, Ramji AF, Hassanzadeh H, Wohlgemut JM, Ain MC, Sponseller PD. Cannulated lag screw fixation of displaced lateral humeral condyle fractures is associated with lower rates of open reduction and infection than pin fixation. J Pediatr Orthop 2017;37(1):7–13

Medial Epicondyle Fracture
1. Farsetti P, Potenza V, Caterini R, Ippolito E. Long-term results of treatment of fractures of the medial humeral epicondyle in children. J Bone Joint Surg Am 2001;83-A(9):1299–1305
2. Josefsson PO, Danielsson LG. Epicondylar elbow fracture in children. 35-year follow-up of 56 unreduced cases. Acta Orthop Scand 1986;57(4):313–315

Elbow Dislocation
1. Carlioz H, Abols Y. Posterior dislocation of the elbow in children. J Pediatr Orthop 1984;4(1):8–12
2. Fowles JV, Kassab MT, Douik M. Untreated posterior dislocation of the elbow in children. J Bone Joint Surg Am 1984;66(6):921–926
3. Nestor BJ, O'Driscoll SW, Morrey BF. Ligamentous reconstruction for posterolateral rotatory instability of the elbow. J Bone Joint Surg Am 1992;74 (8):1235–1241

Radial Head/Neck Fractures
1. Metaizeau JP, Lascombes P, Lemelle JL, Finlayson D, Prevot J. Reduction and fixation of displaced radial neck fractures by closed intramedullary pinning. J Pediatr Orthop 1993;13(3):355–360
2. Steele JA, Graham HK. Angulated radial neck fractures in children. A prospective study of percutaneous reduction. J Bone Joint Surg Br 1992;74 (5):760–764

Monteggia Fracture Dislocations
1. Bado JL. The Monteggia lesion. Clin Orthop Relat Res 1967;50(50):71–86
2. Foran I, Upasani VV, Wallace CD, et al. Acute pediatric Monteggia fractures: a conservative approach to stabilization. J Pediatr Orthop 2017;37(6):e335–e341

7.5 Pediatric Hand and Wrist Fractures

7.5.1 Distal Radial Physeal Fractures

1. Background:
    a) Distal radius physis opens at 3 to 18 months and closes at 17 to 19 years.
    b) Mechanism: Fall on outstretched hand and wrist.
    c) Radial physeal injuries far more common than ulnar.
    d) Salter I and II fractures most common, but Salter III and IV fractures and triplane possible.
2. Treatment:
    a) Try one or two gentle reductions; if successful, immobilize in neutral position or pronation.
    b) If unreducible, especially Salter III or IV: Open reduction with pinning.
3. Complications:
    a) Compartment syndrome.
    b) Medial nerve injury.
    c) Growth arrest (rare).

7.5.2 Scaphoid Fractures

1. Background and treatment:
    a) Most commonly injured carpal bone with incidence between 12 and 15 years.
    b) May occur with distal radius fracture.
    c) If diagnosis is made within 0 to 3 months, then it will usually heal with a short-arm thumb spica cast.
    d) Delayed union of more than 3 months → bone graft.

7.5.3 Metacarpophalangeal Joint Injuries

1. Background:
    a) Fracture or dislocation.
    b) Collateral ligament does not protect physis of proximal phalanx or metacarpal head.
2. Fracture treatment:
    a) "Extra octave" fracture of small finger:
        1. Reduce using pencil in web space as a fulcrum.
        2. Reduction should be maintained when pressure is released.
        3. Hold with rolled cotton gauze between digits.
    b) Intra-articular fractures:
        1. If fragment is greater than 25% of the joint surface or involves any tendon insertion, it needs to be reduced to within 2 mm of anatomic alignment.
        2. Growth arrest is seen in less than 1% of patients.

3. Dislocations:
   a) Often complex dorsal dislocation:
      1. Volar plate entrapped.
      2. Joint space wide, diaphyses parallel.
      3. Sesamoids interposed.
      4. Skin dimpled on volar surface.
   b) Treatment:
      1. One or two attempts at closed reduction.
      2. Open reduction: Volar or dorsal approach.
      3. Incise superficial transverse ligament lateral to volar plate.

7.5.4 Pediatric Thumb Metacarpal Fractures

1. Background and treatment:
   a) Metaphyseal or Salter I and II fractures: Attempt closed reduction and cast; pin if unacceptable.
   b) Pediatric Bennett fractures: Closed reduction or ORIF if more than 1 mm displacement.
   c) Gamekeeper's fracture.
      1. Stener lesion, usually a Salter III type.
      2. ORIF if displaced more than 1 mm on normal radiographs.
      3. With positive stress test at 45 degrees of flexion.

7.5.5 Phalangeal Shaft Fractures

1. Background and treatment:
   a) Less common in children than in adults.
   b) May accept 10 degrees dorsal/palmar angulation.
   c) Immobilization: Short arm cast/splint.

7.5.6 Phalangeal Neck (Subcondylar) Fractures

1. Background:
   a) Most occur in proximal phalanx.
   b) Volar angulation is the most common.
   c) Minimal remodeling occurs in this region.
2. Treatment:
   a) Closed reduction.
   b) Transarticular percutaneous pinning for 3 weeks.
   c) Buddy-tape for 1 week.
   d) Late presentation: May openly reconstruct up to 4 weeks postfracture.
      1. Malunion: Loss of flexion may occur if malposition with bony impingement is allowed to persist.
      2. Treatment: Volar approach and removal of bony block to flexion.

7.5.7 Distal Phalanx Fractures

1. Background:
   a) Mechanism: Crush, hyperflexion, hyperextension.
   b) Classification:
      1. Extraphyseal: Transverse, cloven-hoof, comminuted.
      2. Physeal.
      3. Dorsal mallet injuries.
2. Treatment:
   a) Clean thoroughly and replace nail under fold.
   b) Closed reduction if displacement minor, otherwise ORIF.
   c) Open reduction is indicated if injury involves avulsion of flexor digitorum profundus.
   d) Follow-up to rule out infection.

Bibliography

1. Crick JC, Franco RS, Conners JJ. Fractures about the interphalangeal joints in children. J Orthop Trauma 1987;1(4):318–325
2. Kozin SH, Waters PM. Fractures and dislocations of the hand and carpus in children. In: Beaty JH, James KR, eds. Rockwood and Wilkins Fractures in Children. 7th ed. Philadelphia, PA: Lippincott Williams and Wilkins; 2010:226–288
3. Simmons BP, Peters TT. Subcondylar fossa reconstruction for malunion of fractures of the proximal phalanx in children. J Hand Surg Am 1987;12 (6):1079–1082
4. Waters PM. Operative carpal and hand injuries in children. J Bone Joint Surg Am 2007;89(9):2064–2074

7.6 Pediatric Spine Fractures

7.6.1 Cervical Spine Fractures

1. General principles:
   a) The child should be transported on a special backboard to accommodate large head: recess under head or lift under shoulders.
   b) Obtain radiographs if:
      1. Unconscious patient.
      2. Neck pain.
      3. Head or facial bruising in motor vehicle accident.
   c) Recommended films:
      1. Lateral, anteroposterior, open mouth.
      2. Oblique only if dislocation or subluxation is suspected.

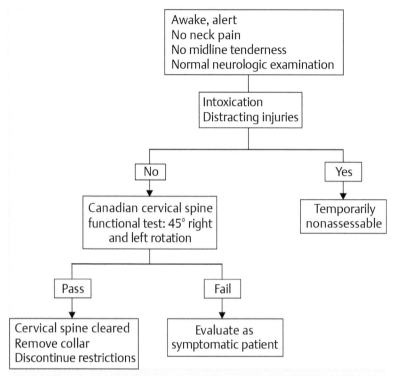

Fig. 7.12 Evaluation of the asymptomatic blunt trauma patient. (Used with permission from Anderson PA, Gugala Z, Lindsey RW, Schoenfeld AJ, Harris MB. Clearing the cervical spine in the blunt trauma patient. J Am Acad Orthop Surg 2010; 18(3):149–159 (Fig. 1).)

d) Normal values (see Chapter 1 [Fig. 1.15]).
e) Algorithms are shown for "clearing" (ruling out injury) in the trauma patient with normal radiographs but with tenderness or altered consciousness (▶ Fig. 7.12; ▶ Fig. 7.13; ▶ Fig. 7.14; ▶ Fig. 7.15).
2. Atlanto-occipital displacement (▶ Fig. 7.16):
   a) Usually skull is distracted and displaced forward. Suspect if dens–basion distance is greater than 12 mm or occipital condyles are not resting in the superior facets of the atlas, or the Power ratio is greater than 1. Confirm with CT or MRI. Document neurologic status.
   b) Immobilize with recessed backboard and minimal or no traction.
   c) Fusion of occiput to C1 or C2 is the most commonly accepted treatment.

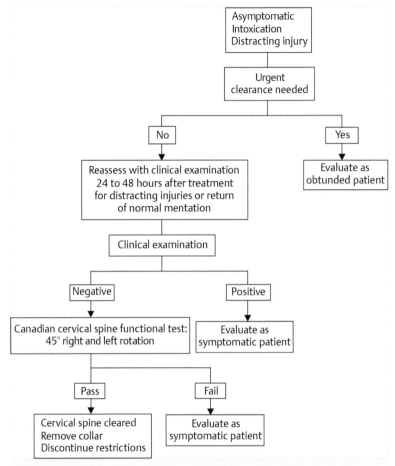

Fig. 7.13 Evaluation of the temporarily unassessable trauma patient. (Used with permission from Anderson PA, Gugala Z, Lindsey RW, Schoenfeld AJ, Harris MB. Clearing the cervical spine in the blunt trauma patient. J Am Acad Orthop Surg 2010;18(3):149–159 (Fig. 2).)

3. Odontoid fracture: reduce and hold in halo or Minerva brace for 8 weeks; then a Philadelphia collar for 4 weeks.
4. Atlas (C1 or Jefferson) fracture:
   a) Minimum (< 7 mm) spread of lateral masses → Philadelphia collar.
   b) If significant spread of lateral masses (> 7 mm) is seen, then traction for 4 weeks followed by collar.

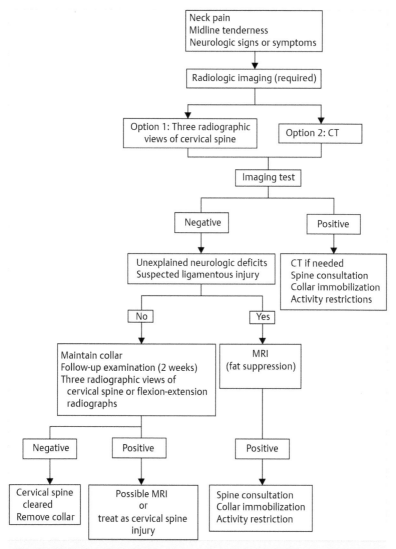

Fig. 7.14 Evaluation of the symptomatic trauma patient. (Used with permission from Anderson PA, Gugala Z, Lindsey RW, Schoenfeld AJ, Harris MB. Clearing the cervical spine in the blunt trauma patient. J Am Acad Orthop Surg 2010;18(3):149–159 (Fig. 3).)

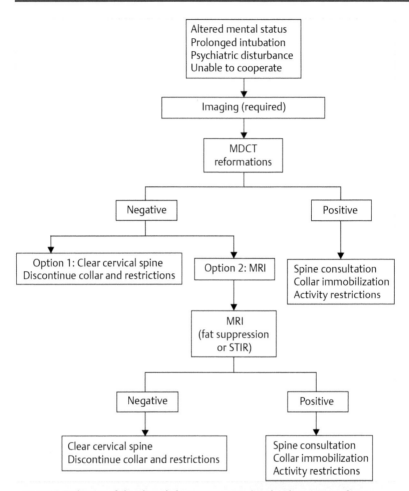

Fig. 7.15 Evaluation of the obtunded trauma patient. (Used with permission from Anderson PA, Gugala Z, Lindsey RW, Schoenfeld AJ, Harris MB. Clearing the cervical spine in the blunt trauma patient. J Am Acad Orthop Surg 2010;18(3):149–159 (Fig. 4).)

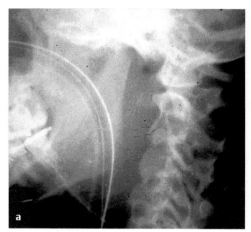

Fig. 7.16 (a,b) Atlanto-occipital displacement.

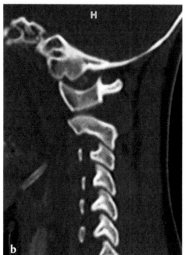

5. C1–C2 rotatory subluxation (▶ Fig. 7.17):
   a) CT scan is the best study to confirm diagnosis.
   b) Symptom duration less than 1 week → collar, analgesics, bed rest, exercises to reduce.
   c) Symptom duration longer than 1 week → halter traction.
   d) Symptom duration longer than 1 month → halo traction, attempt reduction. Fuse in situ if not reducible.

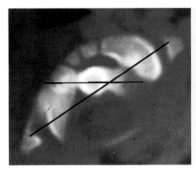

Fig. 7.17 C1–C2 rotatory subluxation.

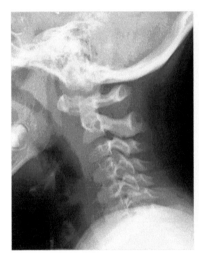

Fig. 7.18 Transverse ligament insufficiency.

6. Transverse ligament insufficiency or os odontoideum (▶ Fig. 7.18): Assess with flexion–extension views.
   a) 3 to 4 mm: Normal.
   b) 4 to 8 mm: Collar, restrict activities.
   c) More than 8 mm or any neurologic abnormalities → posterior fusion C1–C2.
7. C2 pedicle fracture (hangman's fracture):
   a) If C2–C3 disk is intact, immobilize in collar or halo.
   b) If C2–C3 disk disrupted, consider anterior spine fusion.

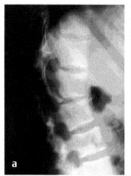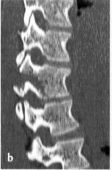

Fig. 7.19 (a,b) Flexion–distraction (chance; seatbelt) injury.

7.6.2 Thoracic and Lumbar Spine Fractures

1. Compression fracture:
   a) If less than 20%, mobilize as tolerated.
   b) If greater than 20%, thoracolumbar spinal orthosis for comfort; mobilize as tolerated.
2. Burst fractures:
   a) If neurologically normal, cast 6 to 8 weeks and then mobilize as tolerated.
   b) If neurologic deficit is present, decompress anteriorly or posteriorly and fuse.
3. Flexion distraction (chance; seatbelt) injuries (▶ Fig. 7.19):
   a) Posterior elements distracted through facets, lamina, or pedicles. Minimal to no compression anteriorly.
   b) Treatment: Attempt reduction in extension and immobilize for 6 to 8 weeks.
   c) If reduction is not obtained or is still unstable or if significant abdominal injury exists, then fuse.

7.7 Pediatric Pelvis and Femur Injuries

7.7.1 Proximal Femur Fractures

1. Background:
   a) Femoral neck physis appears at 4 months; contributes 30% of femur growth.
   b) Mechanism: High-energy trauma; breech delivery in newborns.
2. Delbet classification:
   a) Type I: Transphyseal.
   b) Type II: Transcervical.

c) Type III: Cervicotrochanteric.

d) Type IV: Intertrochanteric.

3. Treatment:

   a) Types I, II, and III are surgical emergencies. Immobilize with cannulated screws. Can use Kirchner wires in Type I.

   b) Type IV: Use dynamic hip screw.

4. Complications:

   a) Avascular necrosis, more likely in Types I and II.

   b) Coxa vara if greater trochanter apophysis is damaged.

   c) Leg-length discrepancy.

7.7.2 Subtrochanteric Fractures

1. Background:

   a) Overgrowth of about 1 cm occurs between ages 2 and 10 years.

   b) One can accept angulation of 25 degrees in any plane.

   c) Fracture tends to develop anterior bow.

   d) Fracture is harder to image in cast.

2. Treatment:

   a) ORIF, plate.

   b) External fixator.

   c) Traction for 3 weeks in 90-degree flexion, then spica cast in 90 degrees of flexion: Be watchful for Volkmann contracture and compartment syndrome with 90 to 90 casts.

7.7.3 Femoral Shaft Fractures

1. Background:

   a) Mechanism: Pedestrian struck by car; fall or sports; passenger in motor vehicle accident.

   b) Overgrowth of about 1 cm occurs between ages 2 and 10 years.

   c) Acceptable reduction: Varus/valgus of up to 10 degrees, anterior/posterior bow of 20 degrees.

   d) Family factors are important in choosing treatment.

   e) Consider child abuse if patient is younger than 2 years.

   f) Hip spica cast is not a good way to maintain length.

2. Treatment:

   a) Age less than 6 years: Does resting overlap less than 2 cm or telescope test show less than 3 cm of shortening?

   1. Yes → spica cast.

   2. No → traction (in hospital or at home) or external fixator.

   b) Age 6 to 10 years:

   1. Flexible intramedullary rods/plate/fixator.

   2. Traction: In hospital or at home.
   3. If resting overlap is less than 2 cm or telescope test shows less than 3 cm of shortening, then a spica cast is an option if the parents so choose.
  c) Age greater than 10 years:
   1. Intramedullary rod with careful preparation of entry hole to avoid disrupting vessels at femoral neck (trochanteric entry).
   2. External fixator.
   3. Plate.
3. Time to union (mean):
  a) Infant: Less than 4 weeks.
  b) Age 2 to 4 years: 4 to 6 weeks.
  c) Age 4 to 6 years: 6 weeks.
  d) Age 6 to 8 years: 6 to 8 weeks.
  e) Times are longer for open or high-energy injuries.

Bibliography

1. Colonna PC. Fractures of the neck of the femur in children. Am J Surg 1929;6:793–797
2. Kanlic E, Cruz M. Current concepts in pediatric femur fracture treatment. Orthopedics 2007;30(12):1015–1019
3. Mubarak SJ, Frick S, Sink E, Rathjen K, Noonan KJ. Volkmann contracture and compartment syndromes after femur fractures in children treated with 90/90 spica casts. J Pediatr Orthop 2006;26(5):567–572

7.8 Physeal Injuries About the Knee

7.8.1 Normal Anatomy and Growth

1. Length of lower limbs doubles between 4 years and maturity.
2. Distal femoral physis:
  a) Quadripod shape.
  b) Ligaments concentrate stress on this physis.
  c) Growth is 1 cm/year until age 13½ (girls), 15½ (boys).
  d) Blood supply to physis comes from epiphyseal vessels primarily, with some contribution from periosteal vessels.
3. Proximal tibial physis:
  a) An anterior extension continues down to the tubercle.
  b) Ligaments, fibula, and semimembranosus insertion protect physis.
  c) Growth is 8 mm/year.

7.8.2 Distal Femoral Physeal Fracture

1. Background:
   a) Most common physeal injury about the knee.
   b) Mechanism: Hyperextension or valgus trauma.
   c) Check for hemarthrosis, especially in Salter III, IV.
   d) May be missed in polytrauma patient.
   e) Ligamentous injury may coexist.
2. Radiographs:
   a) Oblique and tunnel views if needed.
   b) Stress view if occult fracture suspected.
   c) Plain tomograms or CT for complex Salter types III and IV if fracture pattern or displacement is in question.
   d) When to obtain arteriogram:
      1. If vascular examination is abnormal.
      2. Proximal tibia physeal fracture.
      3. Incidence of vascular injury ≤ 1%.
      4. In most cases, arteriogram is not necessary; especially in varus/valgus injuries. Instead, check circulation before and after reduction and instruct caregivers in monitoring it.
3. Treatment:
   a) Gentle closed reduction: One may accept 5 degrees varus/valgus in Salter types I and II.
   b) Open reduction if irreducibly closed.
   c) Pin if unstable.
   d) ORIF all displaced type IV fractures.
   e) Ensure physeal alignment by direct inspection as well as fluoro (at fracture and periphery).
   f) Immobilization:
      1. Long-leg cast if limb is slender and fracture is stable.
      2. Spica cast otherwise.
   g) Begin range of motion by 6 weeks: Follow-up at least 1 year to rule out growth plate injury.
4. Results:
   a) 25 to 50% has length discrepancy greater than 1 cm.
   b) 25% has angular deformity greater than 5 degrees.
5. Treatment of physeal bridge:
   a) Imaging:
      1. Growth lines visible on plain film should be present and parallel to physis if growth is normal.
      2. Tomograms (plain, not CT) if bridge is suspected.
      3. MRI: Discuss with radiologist before study.

b) Indications for resection:
    1. Area of bar is less than 50% of physeal area.
    2. Growth remaining more than 2 years.

7.8.3 Proximal Tibial Physis Injury

1. Background:
    a) One quarter as common as distal femur physeal injury; 5% have popliteal, peroneal injuries.
    b) Mechanism: hyperextension, valgus trauma; 50% occur in sports.
2. Treatment:
    a) Closed versus open reduction; based on standard criteria.
    b) Close vascular monitoring.

7.8.4 Tibial Tubercle Fractures

1. Background:
    a) Many have history of Osgood–Schlatter lesion.
    b) Frequency in males is greater than in females.
    c) Usual age range is 14 to 16 years.
    d) Almost always seen in jumping sports.
2. Treatment:
    a) Closed if minimally displaced and patient can actively extend knee.
    b) ORIF:
        1. Clear bed of interposed tissue.
        2. Use screw if fragment is large and the patient is near maturity.
        3. Otherwise, suture tendon and periosteum.
3. Complications (rarely seen):
    a) Recurvatum: Only if patient is very young (i.e., younger than 11 years).
    b) Lack of flexion.

Bibliography

1. Burkhart SS, Peterson HA. Fractures of the proximal tibial epiphysis. J Bone Joint Surg Am 1979;61(7):996–1002
2. Christie MJ, Dvonch VM. Tibial tuberosity avulsion fracture in adolescents. J Pediatr Orthop 1981;1(4):391–394
3. Flynn JM, Schwend RM. Management of pediatric femoral shaft fractures. J Am Acad Orthop Surg 2004;12(5):347–359
4. Hedequist D, Bishop J, Hresko T. Locking plate fixation for pediatric femur fractures. J Pediatr Orthop 2008;28(1):6–9
5. Ogden JA, Tross RB, Murphy MJ. Fractures of the tibial tuberosity in adolescents. J Bone Joint Surg Am 1980;62(2):205–215
6. Riseborough EJ, Barrett IR, Shapiro F. Growth disturbances following distal femoral physeal fracture-separations. J Bone Joint Surg Am 1983;65(7):885–893

7.9 Physeal Injuries About the Ankle

7.9.1 Background

1. Normal growth:
   a) Distal tibial and fibular epiphyses appear at around the age of 2 years and close between age 12 and 16 years in girls and 14 and 19 years in boys.
   b) The pattern of closure begins centrally, followed by anteromedial, posteromedial, posterolateral, and anterolateral closure.
   c) Distal fibular physis is normally at the level of the tibial plafond.

7.9.2 Fracture Classification (Dias–Tachdjian)

1. Supination–external rotation (SER).
2. Pronation–external rotation.
3. Supination–plantar flexion.
4. Supination–inversion.

7.9.3 Nonarticular Physeal Fractures

1. Closed versus open reduction: Standard criteria (5 degrees varus/valgus is acceptable).
2. Check rotation radiographically and clinically by thigh–foot angle.
3. Use long-leg cast in most cases if displaced.

7.9.4 Tillaux Fractures

1. Background:
   a) Salter–Harris III on anteroposterior.
   b) Anterior inferior tibiofibular ligament avulses unfused epiphyseal fragment.
   c) Mechanism: SER
2. Treatment: Reduce with internal rotation gap greater than 2 mm → ORIF.

7.9.5 Triplane Fracture

1. Background:
   a) Coronal fracture through posterolateral metaphysis, axial fracture through physis, and sagittal fracture through epiphysis (▶ Fig. 7.20):
      1. Most occur as physis starts to close.
      2. Often has appearance of Salter–Harris III on anteroposterior and Salter–Harris II or IV on lateral.
   b) Mechanism: Usually SER at the time of partial closure of physis.

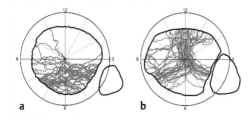

Fig. 7.20 Cross-sectional map of common fracture lines in metaphysis (**a**) and epiphysis (**b**) of triplane fracture.

c) 5 to 10% of pediatric intra-articular distal tibia fractures.
d) There may be two, three, or four parts to the fracture.
e) Concern is mainly articular congruity rather than growth remaining (because most patients with this fracture are nearing maturity).

2. Treatment:
   a) Attempt closed reduction and get CT afterward to confirm.
   b) ORIF if more than 2-mm spread or any vertical displacement.
   c) Anterolateral incision: Reduce posterolateral fragment first, then medial incision if needed.

7.9.6 Salter IV

Reduce and fix if there is any longitudinal displacement or more than 2-mm spread.

7.9.7 Physeal Arrest

1. Distal tibia is the third most common site of growth arrest after fracture:
   a) Represents 25% of all physeal bars.
   b) May occur with Salter type II as well as types III, IV, and V.
2. Implications:
   a) Counsel family of this risk at the time of fracture.
   b) Follow up for a year or longer after injury.
3. Partial arrest:
   a) Calculate potential angulation based on growth remaining.
   b) Some guidelines:
      1. 8 mm = 10-degree deformity will occur if bar forms before age 13½ (boys) or 11½ (girls).
      2. 1-cm growth remains after age 13 (boys), age 11 (girls).
      3. Refer to growth remaining chart (see Chapter 1 [Fig. 1.25]).
4. Bar resection versus epiphysiodesis:
   a) Epiphysiodesis is simpler and more predictable.
   b) Patient's choice.

c) There is less need to do resection than in other areas of the skeleton because length considerations are lessened.

Bibliography

1. Cooperman DR, Spiegel PG, Laros GS. Tibial fractures involving the ankle in children. The so-called triplane epiphyseal fracture. J Bone Joint Surg Am 1978;60(8):1040–1046
2. Crowder C, Austin D. Age ranges of epiphyseal fusion in the distal tibia and fibula of contemporary males and females. J Forensic Sci 2005;50(5):1001–1007
3. Dias LS, Giegerich CR. Fractures of the distal tibial epiphysis in adolescence. J Bone Joint Surg Am 1983;65(4):438–444
4. Feldman F, Singson RD, Rosenberg ZS, Berdon WE, Amodio J, Abramson SJ. Distal tibial triplane fractures: diagnosis with CT. Radiology 1987;164 (2):429–435
5. Kärrholm J, Hansson LI, Selvik G. Longitudinal growth rate of the distal tibia and fibula in children. Clin Orthop Relat Res 1984;191(191):121–128
6. Khoshhal KI, Kiefer GN. Physeal bridge resection. J Am Acad Orthop Surg 2005;13(1):47–58
7. Kling TF Jr, Bright RW, Hensinger RN. Distal tibial physeal fractures in children that may require open reduction. J Bone Joint Surg Am 1984;66 (5):647–657
8. Schnetzler KA, Hoernschemeyer D. The pediatric triplane ankle fracture. J Am Acad Orthop Surg 2007;15(12):738–747

8 Normal Values and Medications

Paul D. Sponseller and Matthew J. Hadad

8.1 Introduction

This chapter includes laboratory values and medications the pediatric ortho-paedic surgeon must know. Pediatric dosages for medication must be calculated based on body weight. Normal laboratory values vary according to age. When giving agents that affect respiration, a plan should also be in place for monitoring and treatment of any adverse responses.

8.2 Normal Laboratory Values (▶ Table 8.1 and ▶ Table 8.2)

Table 8.1 Normal CBC by age

Age	HCT (%) Mean—2 SD	WBC/mm × 100 Mean ± 2 SD (normal ranges)
Newborn	51 (42)	18.1 (9–30)
6 mo	36 (31)	11.9 (6–17.5)
6–24 mo	36 (33)	10.6 (6–17)
2–6 y	37 (34)	8.5 (5–15.5)
>6 y	40 (35)	8.1 (4.5–13.5)

Abbreviations: CBC, complete blood count; HCT, hematocrit; SD, standard deviation; WBC, white blood cell count.

Table 8.2 Normal lab values by age

Parameter	Normal values
Sodium	135–145 mg/dL
Potassium	3.5–5.0 mg/dL
Phosphorus	8–10.5 mg/dL
Alkaline phosphatase	
• Infant	150–400 U/L
• 2–10 y	100–300 U/L
• 11–18 y (male)	50–375 U/L
• 11–18 y (female)	30–300 U/L
• Erythrocyte sedimentation rate	1–5 mm/h
Creatinine	
• Infant	0.2–0.4 mg/dL
• Child	0.3–0.7 mg/dL
• Adult	0.5–1.0 mg/dL
Glucose	
• 1 wk to 16 y	60–105 mg/dL
• >16 y	70–115 mg/dL
Albumin	
• 3–4 mo	2.8–5.0 mg/dL
• 1 y	3.5–5.0 mg/dL
• 2 y to adult	3.3–5.8 mg/dL
ALT (SGPT)	
• <1 y	<54 U/L
• >1 y	1–30 U/L
AST (SGOT)	
• <1 y	25–75 U/L
• >1 y	0–40 U/L

Abbreviations: ALT, alanine aminotransferase; AST, aspartate aminotransferase; SGOT, serum glutamic-oxaloacetic transaminase; SGPT, serum glutamic–pyruvic transaminase.
Source: The Harriet Lane Handbook, 1994.

8.3 Antibiotics (▶ Table 8.3)

Table 8.3 Antibiotic guidelines

Name	Dose	Interval	Route	How supplied	Comments
Amikacin	15–22 mg/kg/d	q8h	i.v., i.m.	Inj. 250 mg/mL	Peak 20–40 µg/mL, trough 5–10 µg/mL
Amoxicillin	Child: 20–50 mg/kg/d	q8h	p.o.	Drops: 50 mg/mL; suspension: 125, 250 mg/mL	Less GI irritation than ampicillin
	Adult: 250–500 mg/dose	q8h	p.o.	Caps: 250, 500 mg; chewable: 125, 250	
Amoxicillin and clavulanic acid (Augmentin)	Child: 20–40 mg/kg/d (approx.)	q8h	p.o.	Suspension: 125 and 250 mg/mL; tabs: 250–500 mg	Used with influenza, *Staphylococcus aureus*, β lactamase producers
Ampicillin	100–400 mg/kg/d	q6h	p.o./i.m./i.v.	Drops: 100 mg/mL; suspension: 125, 250, 500 mg/ml	Maximum oral dose 4 g daily; may cause nephritis
Azithromycin	5–12 mg/kg/dose	q.d.	p.o., i.v.	Tablets: 250–500 mg; solution 500 mg	
Aztreonam	30 mg/kg/dose	q6–8h	i.m., i.v.	Solution: 20–40 mg/mL	
Carbenicillin	400–600 mg/kg/d	q6h	p.o./i.m., i.v. (cut dose to ½)		

Table 8.3 (continued)

Name	Dose	Interval	Route	How supplied	Comments
Cefaclor (Ceclor)	40 mg/kg/d child	q8h	p.o.		Use with caution in renal impaired or pen allergy
Cefadroxil (Duricef, Ultracef)	Child: 30 mg/kg/d	q12h	p.o.		
	Adult: 500–1,000 mg/d				
Cefamandole	Child: 50–150 mg/kg/d	q4–6h	i.m., i.v.		
	Adult: 4–12 g/d				
Cefoperazone (Cefobid)	Child: 100–200 mg/kg/d	q12h	i.m., i.v.		
	Adult: 2–4 g/d				
Cefazolin (Ancef, Kefzol)	Child: 50–100 mg/kg/d	q6–8h	i.m., i.v.		Use with caution in renal failure or pen allergy
Cefdinir	Child: 14 mg/kg/d	q12h or q. d.	p.o.	Capsule: 300 mg	
	Adult: 300 mg	q12h			
Cefepime (Maxipime)	50 mg/kg/dose	q8–12h	i.m., i.v.	Solution: 20 mg/ mL; injection 1–2 g	
Cefotaxime (Claforan)	Child: 100–200 mg/kg/d	q6–8h	i.m., i.v.		
	Adult: 2–12 g/d				
Cefotetan (Cefotan)	Child: 30–50 mg/kg/ dose	q12h	i.m., i.v.	Inj: 1–2 g; IV: 1–2 g	
	Adult: 1–2 g	q12h			

Table 8.3 (continued)

Name	Dose	Interval	Route	How supplied	Comments
Cefoxitin (Mefoxin)	Child: 80–160 mg/kg/d	q4–6h	i.m., i.v.		
	Adult: 4–12 g/d				
Ceftazidime (Fortaz/Ceptaz)	Child: 90–150 mg/kg/d	q8–12h	i.m., i.v.		
	Adult: 2–6 g/d				
Ceftizoxime	Child: 150–200 mg/kg/d	q8h	i.m., i.v.		
	Adult: 2–12 g/d				
Ceftriaxone (Rocephin)	Child: 50–75 mg/kg/d	q12–24h	i.m., i.v.		
	Adult: 1–4 g/d				
Cefuroxime (Zinacef)	Child: 75–150 mg/kg/d	q8h	i.m., i.v.		
	Adult: 2–4.5 g/d				
Cephalexin (Keflex)	Child: 25–50 mg/kg/d	q6h	p.o.	Drops: 100 mg/mL; suspension: 125, 250 mg/5 mL; tabs: 250, 500, 1,000 mg; caps: 250, 500 mg	
	Adult: 1–4 g/d				
Cephalothin (Keflin)	Child: 80–160 mg/kg/d	q4–6h	i.m., i.v.		
	Adult: 2–12 g/d				
Chloramphenicol	50–100 mg/kg/d	q6h	p.o., i.v.		Monitor levels in infants
Ciprofloxacin (Cipro)	500–750 mg	b.i.d.	p.o.		Not recommended in younger than 16 y
	200–400 mg	q2h	i.v.		

Table 8.3 (continued)

Name	Dose	Interval	Route	How supplied	Comments
Clindamycin	Child: 20–30 mg/kg/d	q.i.d	p.o.	Caps: 75, 150, 300 mg	May cause pseudomembranous colitis
	25–40 mg/kg/d	q8–8h	i.m., i.v.	Suspension: 75 mg/5 mL	
	Adult: 600–1,800 mg/d	q6–8h	p.o.		
	600–3,600 mg/d	q6–12h	i.m., i.v.		
Cloxacillin (Tegopen)	Child: 50–100 mg/d	q.i.d.	p.o.	Caps: 250, 500 mg; solution: 125 mg/5 mL	
	Adult: 1–4 g/d				
Daptomycin (Cubicin)	Child 1–5 y old: 10 mg/kg/dose	q.d.	i.v.	IV solution: 500 mg	Avoid use in patients <12 mo for musculoskeletal and neuro adverse effects
	Child 6–11 y old: 7 mg/kg/dose				
	Child 12 to adolescent: 4–6 mg/kg/dose				
	Adult: 4 mg/kg/dose				
Dicloxacillin	Child: 50–100 mg/kg/d	q.i.d.	p.o.		
	Adult: 500–2,500 mg/d	q.i.d.	p.o.		
Doxycycline	5 mg/kg/d	q12h	p.o., i.v.	Caps/tabs: 50, 100; suspension: 25 mg/5 mL	Do not use in children <8 y

Table 8.3 (continued)

Name	Dose	Interval	Route	How supplied	Comments
Ertapenem (Invanz)	Infant and Child: 15 mg/kg/dose	q12h	i.m., i.v.	Solution: 1 g	Administer with cilastatin
	Adolescent and adult: 1,000 mg/d	q.d.			
Erythromycin	Child: 30–50 mg/kg/d	q6–8h	p.o., i.v.		Multiple GI discomfort; give after meals; caution with liver disease
Ethambutol	Adult: 1–4 g/d	q6h	p.o., i.v.		Do not use in children <12 y
	15–25 mg/kg/d	q.d.	p.o.		
Gentamicin	Child: 6–7.5 mg/kg/d	q8h	i.v.		Monitor levels: peak 6–10 mg/L; trough 2 mg/L
	Adult: 3–5 mg/kg/d				
Linezolid (Zyvox)	Children <12 y old: 10 mg/kg/dose	q8h	p.o., i.v.	Tablet: 600 mg; solution, IV: 2 mg/mL; oral suspension: 20 mg/mL	Can cause bone marrow suppression and thrombocytopenia
	Children >12 y old and adults: 600 mg/dose	q12h			
Meropenem (Merrem)	Child: 20 mg/kg/dose	q8h	i.v.	Solution: 500 mg	Maximum dose 1,000 mg/dose
	Adult: 500–2,000 mg/dose	q8h			
Methicillin	Child: 100–400 mg/kg/d	q4–6h	i.m., i.v.		
	Adult: 4–12 g/d				

Table 8.3 (continued)

Name	Dose	Interval	Route	How supplied	Comments
Metronidazole (Flagyl)	Load with 15 mg/kg, then 7.5 mg/kg/dose	q6h	i.v.		
Oxacillin	Child: 50–100 mg/kg/d	q6h	i.v., p.o.		
	Adult: 500–1,000 mg/dose		p.o.		
Penicillin G	Child: 100,000–4000,000 unit/kg/d	q4–6h	i.v.		Probenecid may prolong
	25–50 mg/kg/d	q6–8h	p.o.		
	Adult: 2–24 million unit/d	q4–6h	i.v.		
	125–500 mg/dose	q6h	p.o.		
Penicillin G (potassium)	Child: 25–05 mg/kg/24 h	q6h	p.o.		Must be taken 1 h before or 2 h after meals
	Adult: 250–500 mg/dose	q6h	p.o.		
Piperacillin-tazobactam (Zosyn)	Children > 9 mo: 100 mg piperacillin/kg/dose	q8h	i.v.	Solution: 2 g piperacillin with 0.25 g tazobactam	Maximum dose 16 g piperacillin/d
	Adult: 3,000 mg piperacillin/dose	q6h			
Rifampin	0–20 mg/kg/dose	q12–24h	i.v., p.o.		Colors secretions red

Table 8.3 (continued)

Name	Dose	Interval	Route	How supplied	Comments
Trimethoprim–Sulfamethoxazole (Bactrim)	Child: 6–12 TMP/kg/d	q12h	p.o., i.v.		
	Adult: 160–320 mg Trimethoprim	q12h or q.d.	p.o.		
Tetracycline HCL	Adult: 8–20 mg TMP/kg/d	q6–12h	i.v.		
	Older child: 25–50 mg/kg/d	q6h	p.o.		Do not use in < 8 y
	Adult: 1–2 g/d				
Ticarcillin	200–300 mg/kg/d	q4–6h	i.m., i.v.		Contains Na
Tobramycin	Child: 6–7.5 mg/kg/d	q8h	i.v.		Check levels; peak 6–10 mg/L, trough < 2 mg/L
	Adult: 3–5 mg/kg/d				
Vancomycin	Child: 10 mg/kg/dose	q8h	i.v.		Benadryl can reverse red man syndrome
	Adult: 2 g/d	q8–12h			

Abbreviations: i.m., intramuscular; IV, intravenous; p.o., orally; q.d., every day; q.i.d., four times daily.

8.4 Other Medications Frequently Used in Pediatric Orthopedics (▶ Table 8.4)

Table 8.4 Other medications frequently used in pediatric orthopaedics

Medication	Dose	Interval	Route	Comments/Side effects
Acetaminophen (Tylenol)	65 mg/kg/24 h	q4–6h	p.o./p.r.	Hepatotoxicity; exacerbates g6PD
Acetaminophen + oxycodone (Percocet)	0.1–0.2 mg oxycodone /kg/ dose	q4–6h	p.o.	
Acetaminophen + hydrocodone (Vicodin)	<50 kg: 0.1–0.2 mg hydrocodone/kg/dose	q4–6h	p.o.	
	>50 kg: 5–10 mg hydrocodone	q4–6h	p.o.	
Albuterol (Proventil, Ventolin)	2–5 y: 3 mg/kg/d	q8h	p.o., inhalant nebulizer	Tachycardia
	6–11 y: 2 mg/dose			
	>12 y: 2–4 mg/dose			
Amitriptyline (analgesia)	0.1 mg/kg/dose, may advance as tolerated to 2 mg/kg	q.d.	p.o.	
Ascorbic acid (vitamin C)	35–50 mg/kg	q.d.	p.o.	
Aspirin	65 mg/kg 24 h; max 3–6 g/24 h	q4–6h	p.o./p.r.	GI upset, bleeding. Do not use for chicken pox or flulike symptoms THERAPEUTIC levels 150–300 mg/L
Baclofen	Initial dose 5 mg	t.i.d.	p.o.	Avoid abrupt withdrawal

Table 8.4 (continued)

Medication	Dose	Interval	Route	Comments/Side effects
	Increase 5 mg t.i.d. q3d until maximum of 10–15 mg t.i.d. for child 2–7 y			
	20 mg t.i.d. for child 7–8 y			
	20 mg q.i.d. for adult			
Beclomethasone	1 to 2 inhalations	q6h		
Bisacodyl (Dulcolax)	2–11 y, 5–10 mg	p.r.n.	p.r.	Effect takes 30 min
	>11 y, 10 mg			
Calcium carbonate (Os-Cal, Tums)		q.i.d.	p.o.	May cause constipation
Celecoxib (Celebrex)	10–25 kg: 50 mg/dose	q12h	p.o.	Risk of thrombosis
	>25 kg: 100 mg/dose	q12h	p.o.	
Chloral hydrate—sedative/hypnotic	50–100 mg/kg/dose			
Cimetidine	Children: 20–40 mg/kg/d	q8–12h		Contraindicated in renal, cardiac disease
	Adults: 1.2 g/d			
Codeine	1 mg/kg/dose	q4h	p.o./i.m.	
Coumadin (Warfarin)	Treatment target INR is 2–3; for low-dose prophylaxis, target INR is 1.5–1.9	p.o.		
Dantrolene for malignant hyperthermia crisis	1 mg/kg; repeat until signs and symptoms normalize, up to 10 mg/kg			
Diazepam (Valium)	Sedative: 0.1–0.3 mg/kg/d	q2–4h	i.m./p.o.	
	Anticonvulsant: 0.1–0.3 mg/ kg/dose		i.v. bolus	

Table 8.4 (continued)

Medication	Dose	Interval	Route	Comments/Side effects
	Rate should not exceed 5 mg/min. Maximum dose: infants and toddlers, 5 mg. Older children, 15 mg. May repeat q15 min, ×2			
Diphenhydramine (Benadryl)	Child: 5 mg/kg/d	q6h	p.o., i.v.	
	Adult: 100–200 mg/d	q6h	p.o., i.v.	
Dimetapp (decongestant/antihistamine)	1 mo to 2 y: 1.25 mL	q6–8h	p.o.	
	2–4 y: 3.75 mL	q6–8h	p.o.	
	4–12 y: 5 mL	q6–8h	p.o.	
	>12 y: 5–10 mL	q6–8h	p.o.	
	1 tab	q12h	p.o.	
Docusate sodium laxative (Colace)	<3 y: 10–40 mg/24 h	q6–12h	p.o.	
	3–6 y: 20–60 mg/24 h	q6–12h	p.o.	
	6–12 y: 40–120 mg/24 h	q6–12h	p.o.	
	>12 y: 50–200 mg/24 h	q6–12h	p.o.	
Docusate and casanthranol (laxative) (Peri-Colace)	5–10 mL	q.h.s.	p.o.	
Fentanyl	0.5–3.0 μg/kg/dose	q1h	i.v.	Give over 3 min
Ferrous sulfate	Drops (15 mg Fe/0.6 mL)	q8h	p.o.	
	Syrup (18 mg Fe/5 mL)			
	Elixir (44 mg Fe/5 mL)			
	Tablet (60 mg Fe/tab)			
	Dose 3 mg Fe/kg/24 h			

Table 8.4 (continued)

Medication	Dose	Interval	Route	Comments/Side effects
Folic acid (vitamin)	Dose 1 mg/d		p.o.	
Furosemide (Lasix)	Child: 1 mg/kg/dose (may increase by 1 mg/kg/dose) Adult: 20–80 mg/dose	q6–12h	i.v.	
Haloperidol (sedative)	0.01–0.1 mg/kg	q2h	p.o.	
Hydromorphone (Dilaudid)	1–4 mg	q4–6h	p.o., i.v., i.m.	Fewer side effects than morphine sulfate
Ibuprofen (Motrin, Advil)	20–40 mg/kg/d (suspension = 100 mg/tsp) (tablets = 200, 400, 600 mg)	q6–8h	p.o.	
Ketamine (hypnotic)	4–8 mg/kg		i.m.	May cause laryngospasm, respiratory depression
	0.5–2 mg/kg		i.v.	
Ketorolac (Toradol)	Child: 1 mg/kg load, 0.5 mg/kg dose	q6h	i.v.	Do not use parenterally > 5 d
	Adult: 10 mg	q6h	p.o.	
Lidocaine—local anesthetic	Up to 1 mg/kg for regional block			
Meperidine HCL (Demerol)	Child: 1–1.5 mg/kg/dose	q6h	p.o./i.m./i.v.	
	Adult: 50–150 mg/dose	q6h	p.o./i.m./i.v.	
Methadone (Dolophine)	0.1 mg/kg/dose	q4h for 2–3 doses, then q6–12h as needed	p.o./i.m./i.v.	

Table 8.4 (continued)

Medication	Dose	Interval	Route	Comments/Side effects
Methylprednisolone (steroid dose for spinal cord injury)	30 mg/kg bolus, then 5.4 mg/kg/h × 23 h		i.v.	
Midazolam (sedative/amnestic; Versed)	0.05–0.15 mg/kg/dose	q4h	i.m., s.c.	
	1.0 mg/kg/dose		p.r.	
Morphine sulfate	0.1–0.3 mg/kg/dose	q4h	i.m., s.c.	
	0.1 mg/kg/dose	q2h	i.v.	
Naloxone (Narcan)	Continuous: 0.025–2 mg/kg/h			Short acting, may need redose
	0.01–0.1 mg/kg/dose			
	Up to maximum 2 mg/dose. Repeat q 3–5 min			
Naproxen (Aleve)	10 mg/kg/d (suspension = 125 mg/tsp) (tablets 250 and 375 mg)	q12h	p.o.	
Nortriptyline (analgesia)	Titrate up to 0.05–1 mg/kg/dose	q.d.	p.o.	Max dose 3 mg/kg/d or 150 mg/d
Nystatin (antifungal, topical)	Infants: 1 mL	q6h	p.o.	
	Children: 2–3 mL	q6h	p.o.	
Ondansetron (Zofran)	0.15 mg/kg/dose	q4h × 3	i.v.	
Oxycodone (OxyContin)	Child: 0.05–0.15 mg/kg/dose	q6h	p.o.	Abuse potential, urinary retention
Paraldehyde (sedative/hypnotic)	Adult: 5 mg		i.m./p.o./p.r.	
	0.3 mL/kg/dose			

Table 8.4 (continued)

Medication	Dose	Interval	Route	Comments/Side effects
Paregoric (analgesic)	0.25–0.5 mL/kg/dose	q6h	p.o.	
Prochlorperazine (antiemetic; Compazine)	(>2 y only) 0.4 mg/kg/d	q6–8h	p.o./p.r.	
Promethazine (Phenergan)	0.13 mg/kg (single dose)		i.m.	
	Child: 0.25–0.5 mg/kg/dose	q4h	p.o./i.m./i.v.	
Ranitidine HCL (Zantac)	Child: 2–4 mg/kg/d	q12h	p.o.	
	1–2 mg/kg/d	q12h	i.v.	
Tramadol (Ultram)	Child: 1–2 mg/kg/dose up to 100 mg	q4–6h	p.o.	Potential respiratory complications
	Adults: 50–100 mg/dose	q4–6h		
Tranexamic acid	100 mg/kg loading dose followed by 10 mg/kg/h until closure	N/A	i.v.	
Trimethobenzamide (antiemetic; Tigan)	<13.6 kg: 100 mg	q6–8h	p.o.	
	13.6–40 kg: 100–200 mg	q12h	p.o.	
	>40 kg: 300 mg	q12h	p.o.	
Valproate (Depakote, antiepileptic)	Initial 10–15 mg/kg/d, increasing by 5–10 mg/kg/d weekly	q8–24h	p.o.	

Abbreviations: b.i.d., twice daily; GI, gastrointestinal; G6PD, glucose-6-phosphate dehydrogenase; i.m., intramuscular; i.v., intravenous; p.o., orally; p.r., per rectum; q.i.d., four times daily; s.c., subcutaneous.

8.5 Latex Allergy Prevention

8.5.1 Etiology

1. Multiple exposures.
2. Genetic predisposition.

8.5.2 Patients at Risk

1. Myelodysplasia.
2. Exstrophy.
3. Cerebral palsy with shunt.
4. Other congenital urologic anomalies.

8.5.3 Management

Treat acute episodes with epinephrine, bronchodilators, and steroids. But best is to avoid exposure to latex. Latex-containing items include the following:

- Band-Aid bandages.
- Black anesthesia masks.
- Blood pressure cuff and attached tubing.
- Buretrol latex diaphragm.
- Cloth tape.
- Coban dressings.
- Condom catheters (Texas).
- Dental dams.
- Fresh gas flow anesthesia machine tubing.
- Gloves:
  - Baxter exam gloves.
  - Bio Gel D.
  - Brown Milled.
  - Eudermic.
  - Micro-Touch.
  - Neutraderm.
  - Neutralon.
  - Perry Derma-Guard.
  - Pristine.
  - Safeskin.
  - Sensi-Derm.
  - Ultraderm.
- Intravenous tubing injection ports.
- Medication vial stoppers (not considered to be an allergy risk with usual use).

- Nondisposable temperature probes.
- Nuk nipples and some other feeding nipples and pacifiers.
- Penrose drains.
- Red rubber endotracheal tubes.
- Red rubber nasopharyngeal airways (Rusch).
- Red rubber urinary catheters.
- Tourniquets.
- Ventilator bellows (not considered to be an allergy risk with usual use).

Latex-free items include the following:
- 3 M tapes (Microfoam/Micropore).
- Catheters: Ureteral.
- Cautery cords (Olsen, Valley Laboratory).
- Cautery pads (3M).
- Dermaclear/Dermacil tape (Johnson & Johnson).
- Dermaprene.
- Ear tubes (Richard, Xomed).
- Elastyren.
- Hemovac drains (latex inside).
- Jackson-Pratt drains.
- Nellcor oximeter probes.
- Neolon.
- Plastic oral airways.
- Portex nasal airways.
- Safe gloves.
- Salem sump tubes.
- Silicone Foley catheters (Sherwood).
- Silk tape.
- Standard endotracheal tubes (Portex, Mallinckrodt).
- Steri-Strips (3M).
- Suction, Silastic Foley's (argyle, Bard, Surgicath, Mentor).
- Tactylon.
- Tegaderm (3M).
- Ureteral catheter (Surgicath).
- Vessiloops (Devon Industries).
- Vinyl examination gloves.
- Xeroform (Sherwood Medical).

Bibliography

1. Dormans JP, Templeton JJ, Edmonds C, Davidson RS, Drummond DS. Intra-operative anaphylaxis due to exposure to latex (natural rubber) in children. J Bone Joint Surg Am 1994;76(11):1688–1691
2. Emans JB. Allergy to latex in patients who have myelodysplasia. Relevance for the orthopaedic surgeon. J Bone Joint Surg Am 1992;74(7):1103–1109

9 Common Procedures in Pediatric Orthopaedics

Paul D. Sponseller

9.1 Introduction

This chapter covers procedures commonly needed in the daily care of children, including techniques for the application of traction, administration of regional blocks, and aspiration of major joints.

9.2 Skin and Skeletal Traction

9.2.1 Indications for Skin Traction

Skin traction is used in children for conditions that require moderate traction for reduction or comfort. It is limited by the shear resistance of skin, which is about 2 to 4 pounds per limb in younger children and 5 to 7 pounds per limb in older children. If these parameters are exceeded, blisters may form. Skin is also more sensitive when it has been traumatized or when there is swelling from an adjacent fracture. Skeletal traction is an option if skin traction is not suitable. Some indications for skin traction include the following:

1. Treatment of developmental dysplasia of the hip (DDH) up to about age 2 to 3 years.
2. Restoring abduction in stiff, adducted hips with Perthes disease.
3. Femur fractures until definitive fixation or immobilization.
   a) As definitive treatment if a cast is contraindicated and there is no spasticity.
   b) As temporary treatment until definitive stabilization is performed.
4. To promote resolution of transient synovitis.

9.2.2 Skin Traction Application

1. Apply tincture of benzoin (if desired) followed by a single layer of soft roll. Do not apply adhesive traction strips directly to skin. Application of more than a single layer of soft roll would allow traction to slip off when weight is applied.
2. Place an adhesive strip in a sugar tong or **U** shape on the limb as shown in ▶ Fig. 9.1. Be sure to pad the malleoli well. If the traction weight is to approach the limit stated earlier, distribute the shear over the maximum area by bringing the wrap up to the thigh.

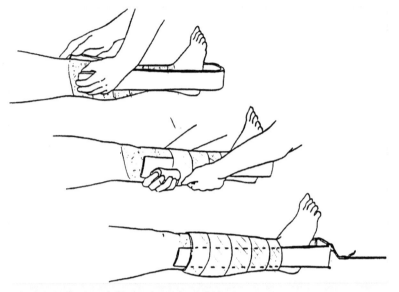

Fig. 9.1 Application of skin traction to lower limb.

3. Roll Ace wrap around leg to hold traction strip in place. Do not roll too tightly.
4. Place spreader in loop of adhesive strip. Make sure the malleoli are free.

9.2.3 Skeletal Traction Pin Placement

1. Collect equipment including Steinmann pin set, hand drill, sterile gloves and towels, Lidocaine, and syringe with needle and scalpel.
2. Inject local anesthetic into the entrance and exit areas, ensuring that the periosteum is thoroughly numb. Femoral nerve block is also an option (see later).
3. Make a small skin incision at the entry site. Use a hemostat to spread the soft tissue down to bone. *Note:* For a femoral pin, enter medially 1 cm above the physis, which is at the adductor tubercle (▶ Fig. 9.2a). For a tibial pin, enter laterally 1 cm distal to and posterior to the base of the tibial tubercle (▶ Fig. 9.2b).
4. Have an assistant stabilize the limb with longitudinal traction and counter pressure. Select a pin and insert it into the entry hole. Feel the anterior and posterior edges of the bone by gently "walking" the pin along the cortex. Determine the midpoint, and press the tip of the pin in. Adjust the angle of the pin to ensure its exit at the proper position. Maintain pressure.

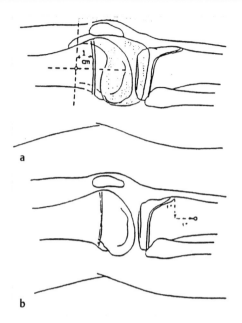

Fig. 9.2 Insertion sites on children for (**a**) femoral pin and (**b**) tibial pin.

a

b

5. Drill through the bone until the pin tents the skin on the far side.
6. Make a small incision to allow the pin to exit the skin. Advance the pin and place traction bow. Cut any sharp ends off the pin and protect.

9.2.4 Traction Assembly

1. Modified Bryant traction: Use for DDH and, rarely, hip fractures for infants (▶ Fig. 9.3). If a higher angle of flexion is desired, a horizontal bar may be used over the top of the crib.
2. Split Russell traction: Use in children with hip synovitis or awaiting treatment of fracture of midshaft of femur (▶ Fig. 9.4). This may be applied as skin or skeletal traction. The hip and knee are flexed 20 to 30 degrees. The term *split* is used because in the original Russell traction, the same weight was used to provide the vertical as well as the longitudinal traction.
3. Ninety-ninety traction (skeletal traction): Use for treatment of femur fractures in children (▶ Fig. 9.5). It is appropriate for fractures of the proximal, midshaft, or distal femur. Greater supervision is required to obtain an accurate radiograph, however.

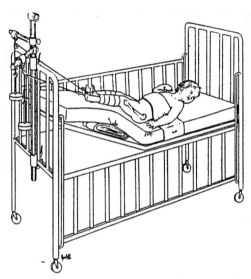

Fig. 9.3 Modified Bryant traction.

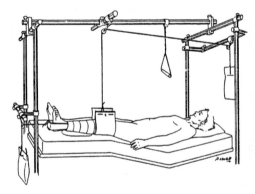

Fig. 9.4 Split Russell traction.

9.2.5 Pediatric Halo and Halo-Vest Application

1. Indications: Use for reduction and immobilization of upper cervical spine fractures and dislocations, such as odontoid fractures, rotatory subluxation, and facet subluxations. Also used for treatment of thoracolumbar spine deformities in preparation for surgery.
2. Technique: Choose halo size so that there is at least 1.5 cm of space between the ring and the cranium circumferentially. Titanium is preferred for magnetic resonance imaging (MRI) compatibility. Stabilize the head while

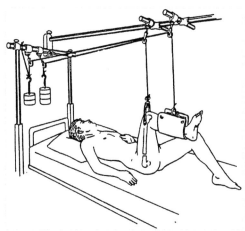

Fig. 9.5 "Ninety-ninety" traction.

obtaining circumferential access by moving to the end of the backboard. Local anesthetic can be injected into desired areas. Systemic analgesia may be given as needed. Anterior pin sites should be 1 cm above the eyebrow and lateral to its midportion to avoid supraorbital and supratrochlear nerves. Posterior pin sites should be diametrically opposite to these. In children younger than 12 years, six to eight pins should be used for increased stability. Torque should be increased incrementally from 2 in-pound at age 2 to 8 in-pound at maturity.

3. If used for traction, weight is increased gradually from approximately 5 pounds initially. Monitor neurologic status at least once per shift, more frequently if weight is increased. This should include check of cranial nerves and upper and lower extremities.

4. Gardner–Wells tongs: These tongs can be used for temporary traction. This assembly consists of two pins, one above each external auditory meatus, inserted until the indicator tab pops out.

9.3 Regional Blocks

9.3.1 Intravenous Regional Anesthesia (Bier Block)

1. Indications: Upper extremity fractures requiring closed reduction but not amenable to single-nerve block.
2. Contraindications:
   a) Fracture above distal humerus.
   b) Vascular injury, compartment syndrome.
   c) Allergy to local anesthetics.
3. Premedication:
   a) Chloral hydrate, 50 to 100 mg/kg either orally or rectally or
   b) Other sedative of choice.
   c) Have available Valium for administration 1 to 2 mg intravenously every 2 minutes as needed for convulsions (incidence < 0.5%).
4. Technique:
   a) Intravenous access in each upper extremity.
   b) Single- or double-cuff tourniquet on upper arm of injured side.
   c) Exsanguinate by gravity for 1 to 2 minutes, then inflate cuff; if double cuff, use most proximal first.
   d) Inflation pressure: 200 to 250 mm Hg.
   e) Inject lidocaine, 0.5%: 0.6 to 1.0 mL/kg (3–5 mg/kg).
   f) Reduce fracture, apply splint or cast, and confirm with radiograph.
   g) If tourniquet pain occurs, change from proximal to distal cuff.
   h) Release: Tourniquet must be up for at least 30 minutes to allow tissue binding of lidocaine.
   i) Deflate tourniquet for a few seconds, then reinflate and repeat over 2 minutes to allow gradual release of anesthetic.

Bibliography

1. Barnes CL, Blasier RD, Dodge BM. Intravenous regional anesthesia: a safe and cost-effective outpatient anesthetic for upper extremity fracture treatment in children. J Pediatr Orthop 1991;11(6):717–720

9.3.2 Axillary Block

1. Indications:
   a) To provide anesthesia for reduction of fractures of the distal humerus or below the hand, wrist, forearm, elbow, distal arm.
   b) For wound debridement, closure, or incision.

2. Contraindications:
   a) Allergy to local anesthetics.
   b) Inability to abduct shoulder.
   c) Bleeding diathesis.
   d) Vascular injury or compartment syndrome.
3. Premedication to decrease anxiety:
   a) Intravenous line in case it is needed.
   b) Children:
      1. Chloral hydrate 50 to 100 mg/kg administered orally or rectally or
      2. Intravenous titration with benzodiazepine/narcotic.
4. Technique of block administration (▶ Fig. 9.6):
   a) Draw up anesthetic agent: Lidocaine or Mepivacaine 5 mg/kg in children, 7 mg/kg in adults (usual adult dose is 40 mL of 1% solution).
   b) Intravenous line and sedation as desired.
   c) Abduct shoulder to about 90 degrees.
   d) Palpate axillary artery, pectoralis and latissimus muscles, and humeral head.
   e) Prepare and drape axilla.
   f) Puncture skin, attempt to puncture axillary artery.
   g) Advance the needle just through the artery with frequent aspiration checks. Inject one-third of the anesthetic agent.
   h) Slowly withdraw the needle to just superficial to the artery, and inject the remainder of the agent, 2 to 3 mL at a time.
   i) Apply direct pressure on the injection site, and fold the extremity across the chest to avoid distal runoff of the solution.
   j) Ultrasound guidance is an option for localization of artery and plexus.

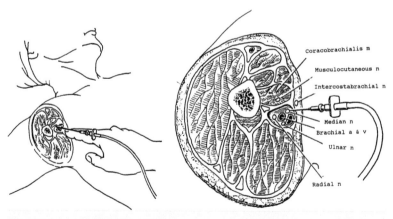

Fig. 9.6 Landmarks for axillary block.

9.3.3 Femoral Nerve Block

1. Indications:
   a) Anesthesia of anteromedial thigh or medial aspect of leg or proximal foot (medial border).
   b) Surgery of anterior thigh: Minor surgery.
   c) Part of multiple lower extremity block for knee and ankle surgery.
   d) Relief of postoperative pain in the knee.
   e) Placement and removal of skeletal traction pins.
   f) Manipulation and reduction of fracture of femur.
2. Contraindications: Ulceration or infection in the groin.
3. Technique:
   a) Draw up anesthetic agent: Lidocaine up to 4 mg/kg or Marcaine (bupivacaine) up to 0.5 mg/kg. Usual adult dose is 20 mL of 1% lidocaine or 10 to 15 mL of 0.5% bupivacaine.
   b) Patient lies supine with thigh on a flat surface.
   c) Landmarks (▶ Fig. 9.7):
      1. The femoral nerve is the most lateral structure in the femoral triangle.
      2. Point of entry: One fingerbreadth lateral to the femoral artery below the inguinal ligament.

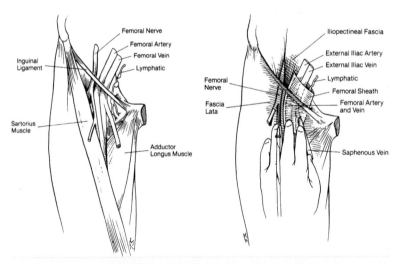

Fig. 9.7 Landmarks for femoral block. Needle insertion is one fingerbreadth lateral to femoral artery. (Used with permission from Pai U, Raj PP. Peripheral nerve blocks. In: Raj PP, ed. Handbook of Regional Anesthesia. New York: Churchill Livingstone; 1985:204.)

d) Insertion:
1. Locally infiltrate the point of entry.
2. Place the middle finger of the nondominant hand on the femoral artery.
3. Insert the needle one fingerbreadth lateral to the artery cephalad at an angle of 30 degrees.
4. Once the position of the needle is confirmed, aspirate for blood.
5. Inject the appropriate volume of local anesthetic.

9.3.4 Popliteal Block

1. Indications: For analgesia during or after procedures on the mid to lower leg or foot. May need to be combined with block of saphenous nerve if complete anesthesia is desired.
2. Technique: Prepare the popliteal region. Flex the knee to determine the outline of medial and lateral hamstring. Ideal location of injection is midway between these two structures, 2 to 3 cm proximal to the knee flexion crease. Use 22- to 25-gauge needle. Aspirate while injecting.

The neurovascular bundle is over two-thirds of the distance between the skin and bone. If blood is obtained, withdraw the needle slightly. Nerve stimulator or ultrasound is a useful adjunct. Inject desired volume (up to 1 mg/kg of bupivacaine if no allergy). Disperse it medially and laterally. Allow at least 20 to 30 minutes for effect. Epinephrine may be used for longer effect if there is no vascular compromise.

9.4 Injection and Aspiration

9.4.1 Technique of Hip Arthrogram/Aspiration

1. Indications:
   a) To assess reduction and morphology of the cartilaginous epiphysis.
   b) To rule out infection.
2. Hip arthrogram with or without aspiration may be performed via anterior, medial, or lateral approach (▶ Fig. 9.8; ▶ Fig. 9.9). An arthrogram is usually performed with any aspiration to verify that the needle is within the joint rather than in other tissue spaces. Ultrasound may also be used.
   Confirmation of joint entry is important before injecting arthrogram dye to avoid extra-articular contrast material obscuring the field. Confirmation is accomplished by three methods:
   a) The sensation of needle popping through the capsule and abutting cartilage (with paradoxical motion on hip rotation).
   b) Radiographic viewing of needle tip (fluoroscopy or ultrasound).
   c) The saline acceptance test.

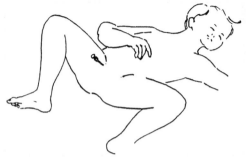

Fig. 9.8 Medial approach for hip aspiration. Needle is inserted just posterior to adductor longus and directed toward anterior superior iliac spine.

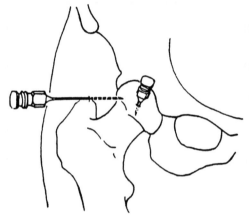

Fig. 9.9 Anterior approach for hip aspiration is two fingerbreadths lateral to the femoral artery, below the inguinal ligament. The lateral approach is just over the tip of the trochanter.

3. Equipment:
   a) Choice of sedation or anesthesia.
   b) Fluoroscope, fluoroscopy table, shields for both doctor and patient, or ultrasound.
   c) Sterile preparation, drape, and gloves.
   d) Needle, 18- to 20-gauge, 1.5 to 3 inches long.
   e) Sterile saline (nonbacteriostatic).
   f) Contrast media.
   g) 10- to 20-mL syringes (two).
   h) Intravenous extension tubing (two).
   i) Cell count and culture tubes if needed.
4. Procedure:
   a) Prepare and drape the area in a fashion that allows the examiner to move the hip during study.

b) Attach syringes to the tubing; fill one with saline, the other with Renografin and label.

c) Localize the skin entry site and needle direction with fluoroscopy. The entry can be anterior, medial, or lateral.

d) Advance the needle until it is felt to pop through the capsule and abut cartilage. There should be paradoxical motion with hip rotation; the needle head should move in the opposite direction of the hip.

e) Confirm location with radiographs.

f) Check for the formation of mucin string on any fluid obtained.

g) Inject 1 to 3 mL of saline. If it flows easily and much of the fluid can be reaspirated, the needle is in the proper location. If much resistance occurs even though needle position is good, it is probably in the femoral head cartilage. If fluid injects easily but does not withdraw, it is probably outside the joint.

h) If joint fluid is to be analyzed and cultured, do it now (before injecting contrast).

i) Detach the saline-filled syringe and tubing; attach a contrast line and use fluoroscopy during initial injection to detect spill early. Inject just enough dye to outline the joint. If closed reduction is to be performed, minimize capsule distention.

j) Obtain motion studies and plain copy radiographs if needed.

k) If the study is being done to rule out infection, it is best done in the fluoroscopy suite with sedation rather than in the operating room. This allows adequate time to analyze joint fluid before deciding on treatment.

9.4.2 Sacroiliac Joint Aspiration or Injection

1. Indications: To rule out infection or to assess the sacroiliac (SI) joint as a site of pain.
2. Equipment:
   a) Fluoroscope, table, gowns.
   b) Needle (18-gauge, 3-inch).
   c) Prepare and drape.
   d) Lidocaine.
   e) Renografin-60.
3. Technique:
   a) The technique described here takes advantage of the relatively simple plane of the distal one-third of the joint.
   b) Turn the patient prone with the unaffected side tilted 10 to 30 degrees up (▶ Fig. 9.10).
   c) Adjust the tilt until the caudal one-third of the affected SI joint is parallel to the beam.
   d) Select the needle entry point using fluoroscopy.

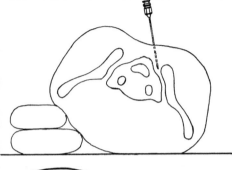

Fig. 9.10 Positioning for aspiration of the sacroiliac joint.

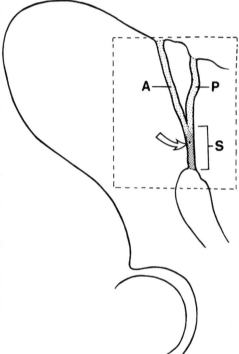

Fig. 9.11 Desired needle placement as seen radiographically. A, anterior; P, posterior; S, straight-ahead. (Used with permission from Hendrix RW, Lin PLP, Kane WJ. Simplified aspiration or injection technique for the sacro-iliac joint. J Bone Joint Surg Am 1982;64(8):1250 (Fig. 1-B).)

e) Infiltrate skin as necessary.

f) Insert needle (3–5 cm for average grown patient), and check for depth with lateral view as needed (▶ Fig. 9.11).

g) Aspirate joint; wash with saline as necessary.

h) Confirm joint entry with contrast.

9.5 Hip Spica Cast Application

9.5.1 Indications

To immobilize a femur fracture or hip dislocation; to immobilize a patient after hip surgery.

9.5.2 Preparation

Pain and motion should usually be controlled by general anesthesia or sedation. Local block (femoral block, above) can be added. Adequate help is needed to control the head and legs; ideally one or two knowledgeable assistants are needed.

Goals are to create proper position of immobilization, adequate room for respiration, wide perineal window, and position of patient for best ease of sitting and transport. Discuss steps and define the position of the cast for which the team should aim.

9.5.3 Equipment

Equipment needed includes a spica table, one or two layers of cast liner or stocking, abundant cast padding, foam or felt for bony prominences, towels to create space for the abdomen, cast material, and cast tape. For infants, waterproof cast material may be used to allow immersion for bathing. Extra cast "splints" are used to reinforce the groin area. A bar between the legs is preferred by some orthopaedists.

9.5.4 Procedure

1. If analgesic block is to be used, do it first.
2. Cast liner or stockinette is applied over the trunk and leg(s). For femur fracture, the foot is most commonly included; for DDH and postoperative cast, the cast may be stopped above the ankle.
3. Foam or felt padding may be applied over SI joints or other prominences (▶ Fig. 9.12a).
4. Patient is positioned on spica table with extra room allowed for the torso portion. Towels may be placed on the abdomen as temporary spacers to allow room for respiration. Legs are held in position of flexion and abduction.
5. For femur fracture, apply the cast in sections. An above-the-knee cast (angle < 90 degrees) is applied to the affected leg with good padding in the popliteal fossa. Cast is applied around the torso as well (▶ Fig. 9.12b). Both are allowed to set.

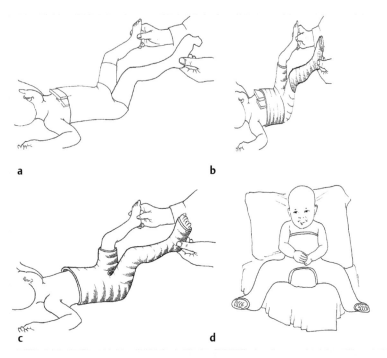

Fig. 9.12 (a–d) Hip spica cast illustrations.

6. Then the reduction of the femur can be performed, maintaining gentle traction and allowing for slight extra valgus. Create narrow medial-to-lateral mold. Add splints across the groin before the final layer because the hip joint of the cast is the weakest area (▶ Fig. 9.12c).

7. For closed reduction of DDH, pay attention to the angle of hip flexion (> 90 degrees) and abduction (for stability and safe zone > 20 degrees). Use padding and molding over affected trochanter(s) to assist reduction.

8. Turn the edges of the cast down. Use tape to hold perineal edges of the liner and create a wide perineal window. Remove towels if used (▶ Fig. 9.12d).

9. Window over abdomen or G-tube if needed.

10. Radiographs or other imaging of hip or femur if indicated.

11. Perform neurologic and vascular checks.

12. Arrange wheelchair and car seat.

9.6 Ponseti Technique for Clubfoot Cast

9.6.1 Indications

The Ponseti technique is indicated for treatment of clubfoot in children younger than 12 to 18 months who have not had surgery. It relies on guided correction of the three-dimensional malrotation of the foot and uses prolonged bracing to maintain the correction during growth. The goal is to avoid operative dissection of the bones of the foot and ankle, which could disturb vascularity and growth and create incongruity. Invasive procedures are minimized and are directed at the tendons as indicated.

9.6.2 Procedures

1. The infant is kept as relaxed as possible, using judicious feeding and minimizing bright light, noise, or other stimuli. Manipulation assesses the components of cavus, adduction, hindfoot varus, and equinus. In bilateral cases, usually one foot is tighter than the other, and this should be noted.
2. Padding is applied, and the foot is held by one worker who is positioned on the lateral side of the foot being treated. The foot is held in the corrected position. Another worker applies the cast of plaster or soft fiberglass. The long-leg cast is applied from the tips of the toes to mid-thigh with the leg flexed 70 to 90 degrees. Avoid changing positions during this stage.
3. Final molding is performed before and during setting of the cast. This involves the following forces:
   a) Dorsiflexion of the first ray, with a finger under the metatarsal head and a thumb over the talar neck to correct the cavus (▶ Fig. 9.13a).
   b) Abduction of the first ray to correct the adduction.
   c) External rotation of the foot to correct the varus.
   d) Gentle dorsiflexion of the ankle.
   e) Mold the above-knee portion of the cast to prevent slipping off.
   f) The cast is changed approximately weekly until the malrotation and adduction are slightly overcorrected (▶ Fig. 9.13b,c). If the hindfoot equinus does not correct beyond neutral into dorsiflexion, an Achilles tenotomy is indicated. This is needed in most cases, usually after three to five cast changes. A stress dorsiflexion lateral radiograph may be obtained if there is any question.
   g) Achilles tenotomy is performed either under local anesthesia in the office (author's preference) or in the operating room with sedation. The Achilles tendon is marked, 1 cm above the calcaneal insertion. It is infiltrated with local anesthetic. After 5 to 10 minutes, it is reprepped and incised with a no. 11 scalpel or Beaver blade. A distinct "give" should be felt. If not, redirect the blade slightly to ensure a complete tenotomy. Bleeding should be controlled with pressure over a sterile dressing. Then a new corrective cast is applied for 2 weeks.

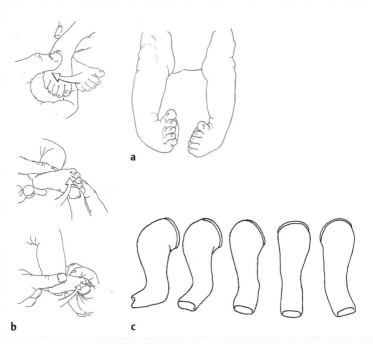

Fig. 9.13 (a–c) Ponseti method for correction of clubfoot.

h) After the last cast, the feet are held in corrected position in a foot abduction orthosis. This is a bar with the feet held in 65 degrees of external rotation and 10 degrees of dorsiflexion on the involved side(s). It is worn full time for 2 months. After that, it is worn at night and nap time for 3 to 5 years, depending on the correction. Compliance with this phase is critical to success of the treatment.

i) During the follow-up phase, a family member should work on stretching the foot into external rotation and eversion and dorsiflexion. As the child matures, instruct on active exercises in these directions.

j) If recurrence is noted, repeat the casting protocol and resume bracing.

k) If residual deformity is noted at around 4 to 5 years, this can usually be corrected by minimally invasive surgery. Equinus can be corrected by an open Achilles tendon lengthening. Internal rotation and adduction can be corrected by transfer of the anterior tibialis tendon to the third cuneiform or base of the third metatarsal. Any fixed deformity should be corrected first.

l) Rarely, resistant cases may require open releases.

9.6.3 Tips and Tricks

1. The fulcrum for the correction involves counter pressure over the talar head, not the calcaneocuboid joint. The goal is to rotate the foot around the talar head and then to dorsiflex it at the tibiotalar joint. Avoid excessive dorsiflexion to prevent flattening of the talar head.
2. If the cast is repeatedly kicked off by the infant, use tincture of benzoin on the skin, increase the degree of knee flexion slightly, and increase the supracondylar molding.
3. If the subcutaneous padding of the foot is thin over the talar head, adhesive padding over this area should be used.
4. If the family is not able to ensure orthosis wear, then meet with them more frequently. Use an interpreter if necessary. Involve other family members if available.
5. One reason for poor tolerance of abduction orthosis is residual deformity. Assess and consider further casting into an overcorrected position.
6. Several varieties of foot abduction orthoses are available. There are foot pieces of soft leather (available through www.mdorthopaedics.com). One design has hinges to allow some kicking movement.
7. If the infant will not tolerate the foot abduction orthosis, then a single-leg knee–ankle–foot orthosis may be ordered that will hold the foot in external rotation and dorsiflexion.

9.7 Minerva Cast Application

9.7.1 Indications

Maintenance of torticollis correction; immobilization of upper cervical spine injuries such as reduced or nondisplaced odontoid fracture.

9.7.2 Equipment

Adequate sedation or analgesia. Cast liner for head. Philadelphia collar to create padded contouring around chin (▶ Fig. 9.14a). Padding for base of neck. Head position can be temporarily maintained using manual support (▶ Fig. 9.14b) or halter (▶ Fig. 9.14c). Hair may need to be trimmed. Thin cast material around the head and neck; wider for torso.

9.7.3 Procedure

Maintain head position using halter or hands. Apply Philadelphia collar around neck. Add cast liner around torso. Apply cast and reinforce around neck. Trim and pad (▶ Fig. 9.14d).

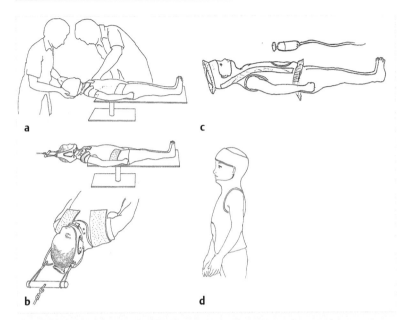

Fig. 9.14 (a–d) Minerva cast illustrations.

Bibliography

1. Hendrix RW, Lin PJ, Kane WJ. Simplified aspiration or injection technique for the sacro-iliac joint. J Bone Joint Surg Am 1982;64(8):1249–1252
2. Jameson SS, Kumar CS. The efficacy of combined popliteal and ankle blocks in forefoot surgery. J Bone Joint Surg Am 2009;91(2):486–487, author reply 487
3. Jarrett GJ, Rongstad KM, Snyder M. Technique tip: popliteal nerve block by surgeon in the lateral decubitus position. Foot Ankle Int 2004;25(1):37–38
4. Miskew DB, Block RA, Witt PF. Aspiration of infected sarco-iliac joints. J Bone Joint Surg Am 1979;61(7):1071–1072
5. Siapkara A, Duncan R. Congenital talipes equinovarus: a review of current management. J Bone Joint Surg Br 2007;89(8):995–1000

Index

Note: Page numbers set **bold** or *italic* indicate headings or figures, respectively.